Tai Chi Walking Exercises for Seniors Over 60

A Complete 28-Day Illustrated Program to Prevent Falls, Rebuild Balance and Walk with Confidence in Just 10 Minutes a Day

Liuhe Chen

Disclaimer

The content in this book is provided for educational purposes and general guidance only. Nothing here replaces a consultation with your doctor or a qualified medical professional. Before starting this seated program or any new form of physical activity, please speak with your physician, especially if you are managing a chronic condition, recovering from injury or surgery, or have recently been unwell.

The author and publisher have taken care to present this material responsibly. Even so, neither accepts liability for any adverse outcome, injury, or loss that may arise from following the guidance in these pages. Use your own judgment, listen to your body, and consult a professional when in doubt.

Table of Contents

A Note from the Author 1

Before You Begin 3

Chapter 1 6

Why Your Walk Changes After 60 6

    What Happens to Your Walking After 60 6

    Why Everyday Walk Doesn't Keep You Safe 8

    Tai Chi Walking Vs. Regular Exercise 9

    Fall Prevention, Balance, and Confidence 11

Chapter 2 13

The Science Behind Safer Steps 13

    How Your Balance System Works 13

    Role of Muscle Memory in Every Step You Take 15

    How Mindful Walking Retrains the Nervous System 16

    Findings on Tai Chi and Fall Prevention 17

Chapter 3 19

Setting Yourself Up for Success 19

    Check In With Your Body Before Each Session 19

    What to Wear, Where to Walk, and What to Avoid 20

    The Warm-Up Routine 21

        Ankle Circles 22

        Knee Bends 23

        Hip Circles 23

        Calf Raises 25

    Your Day One Walking Baseline 25

Chapter 4 27

The Twelve Tai Chi Walking Exercises 27

    How to Read Each Exercise Block 27

        Exercise 1: Grounded Heel Step 27

        Exercise 2: Slow-Motion Forward Walk 29

        Exercise 3: Step and Pause 31

        Exercise 4: Toe-Lift Walk 33

Exercise 5: Wide-Base Side Step 34

Exercise 6: Arm-Swing Coordination Walk 36

Exercise 7: Heel-to-Toe Precision Walk 37

Exercise 8: Figure-Eight Walking Path 38

Exercise 9: Backward Step and Hold 40

Exercise 10: Obstacle Step-Over..41

Exercise 11: Direction-Change Walk 42

Exercise 12: Confidence Walk 43

Common Walking Mistakes Seniors Make – and How to Fix Them 44

Mistake 1: Looking Down at the Feet 44

Mistake 2: Shuffling the Feet...45

Mistake 3: Holding the Arms Stiff..46

Mistake 4: Taking Very Small Steps 46

Mistake 5: Tensing Against a Potential Fall 47

Using a Walking Aid – How to Adapt These Exercises 47

Chapter 5 50

The 28-Day Walking Program 50

Week 1 – Find Your Ground..50

Week 2 – Build Your Balance..55

Week 3 – Walk with Control 59

Week 4 – Walk with Confidence 63

Chapter 6 69

Eating, Resting, and Looking After Your Joints..69

What Your Joints Need to Keep Moving Well 69

Foods That Support Balance and Bone Strength..70

How Rest and Sleep Support Your Walking 71

Managing Pain and Stiffness Between Sessions 72

Chapter 7 75

Walking Safely in the Real World..75

Stairs, Slopes, and Uneven Ground 75

Walking in Busy Places 77

Walking With Confidence After a Fall or a Scare 78

Weather, Lighting, and Outdoor Safety Tips 79

Chapter 8 80

After Day 28 – Keeping the Progress Going...80

Reading Your Day 28 Results Honestly 80

Continuing the Program on Your Own Terms 81

Adding More Distance, Speed, or Challenge 82

Walking for the Long Run 82

Conclusion 85

About the Author 87

A Note from the Author

I want to start with something that most fitness books don't say out loud: worrying about falling is completely reasonable.

Falls are one of the most common and most serious health events for people over 60. They are not just a physical problem. They change how you feel about going out. They change which routes you take, which invitations you accept, and how much you trust your own body. Even a near-fall - a stumble that you caught yourself from - can leave a mark on your confidence that lasts for months.

I have worked with older adults on walking and balance for many years. The single most common thing I hear from people who come to me is some version of this: my walking doesn't feel like it used to. They don't mean they walk slower, though that is often true. They mean something else: the automatic trust they used to have in every step is not quite there anymore. They are thinking about the ground in a way they never had to before.

That change is real, and it has real causes. After 60, several things shift in the way the body manages walking. The muscles that stabilize each step become less reliable. The signals the feet send to the brain about the surface below them become slower and less precise. The time it takes the brain to respond to a sudden change - an uneven paving stone, a threshold between two floors - gets a little longer. None of this is dramatic on its own. Together, these small changes add up to a walk that feels less certain.

Here is the good news: this is not permanent. The body responds to training at any age. The specific kind of training that matters for walking safety is not about fitness in the general sense. It is about teaching the nervous system to manage weight transfer more deliberately, to read the ground more carefully, and to move through each step with more control. That is exactly what Tai Chi walking does.

This program is built around 12 walking exercises drawn from Tai Chi principles. None of them are complicated. None of them require any equipment. You do not need to know anything about Tai Chi before you begin. What you need is a clear floor space, flat comfortable shoes, and about ten minutes each day.

The 28-day program is organized into four weeks, each with a clear focus. Week One is about learning to feel the ground under your feet again. Week Two is about building balance through deliberate weight transfer and side stepping. Week Three brings in the more advanced exercises: precision walking, direction changes, and stepping over obstacles. Week Four puts everything together and applies it to the kind of walking you actually do every day.

There are two rest days in each week, always on the same types of days: a midweek rest and a late-week rest. These are not days off. They are days when the body locks in the work you have done. Skipping them is not more dedicated. It is less effective.

By Day 28, most people who complete this program notice real changes: steadier steps, less hesitation on uneven ground, more confidence going into spaces that used to feel risky. These changes are not magic. They are the result of training the specific systems that walking safety depends on, done consistently, ten minutes at a time.

Start at Chapter Three before Day 1. Take the three baseline assessments. They are short and simple, and they will make your Day 28 results meaningful rather than vague. Then read through Chapter Four before you begin the program, so that when an exercise is mentioned in Chapter Five, you already know what it looks like.

Take your time. Trust the process. The walk you want is built ten minutes at a time.

Liuhe Chen

Before You Begin

A few practical things to sort out before Day 1. None of them take long, and all of them will make the program work better for you.

Talk to Your Doctor First

If any of the following apply to you, please speak with your doctor before starting this program: you have had a fall in the past six months; you have had hip, knee, or ankle surgery in the past year; you have been diagnosed with a condition affecting your balance, such as Parkinson's disease or a vestibular disorder; you have peripheral neuropathy or significantly reduced feeling in your feet; or you have been told by a healthcare provider to limit weight-bearing activity for any reason.

This program uses gentle, slow walking movements. It is one of the lowest-impact exercise programs available for older adults. But walking always involves balance, and balance involves some risk. The safest way to begin is with your doctor's awareness and, where needed, their guidance.

What You Need

Shoes. Flat, well-fitting, non-slip walking shoes. No sandals, no backless shoes, no thick-soled trainers that reduce the feel of the ground underfoot. If you have orthotics, wear them. The shoe should grip the floor lightly but not stick to it.

A clear walking space. You need a straight, unobstructed walking path of at least ten feet for indoor practice. A hallway, a long room with the furniture moved, or an outdoor path on a flat surface all work well. The floor should be non-slip. Avoid thick carpet in the first two weeks while you are learning the exercises.

A sturdy chair nearby. In the early sessions, a chair placed at the edge of your practice space is your safety net. You will not be sitting in it during the exercises, but knowing it is there allows you to practice without bracing against a fall. A dining chair or kitchen chair with four stable legs is ideal. Not a chair on wheels.

That is the full list. No equipment, no technology, no special clothing. Just shoes, space, and a chair within reach. If you have a walking cane or frame, keep it nearby too. The exercises in this book can be adapted for walking aids, and guidance on this is provided at the end of Chapter Four.

How to Use This Book

Read Chapter One and Chapter Two before Day 1. They explain why your walking may have changed, and what this program does about it. Understanding the why behind the exercises helps you get more out of them.

Complete the three baseline assessments in Chapter Three before Day 1. These are simple and take about five minutes. Without them, the progress checks in Chapter Five cannot tell you anything useful about how far you have come.

Read through Chapter Four before you start the program. You do not need to try the exercises yet. You just need to have seen each one at least once, so that when Chapter Five mentions an exercise by name, you know what it looks like.

Chapter Five is the daily program. Each day's entry is short and clear. Read it fully before you start the session, including Liuhe's Note and the NOTICE TODAY prompt. They change the quality of what follows.

Chapters Six, Seven, and Eight support the program. Read Chapter Six during Week Two. Read Chapter Seven during Week Three. Read Chapter Eight after Day 28.

A Word About Rest Days

There are two rest days per week in this program, eight rest days in total. They appear on Day 3, Day 6, Day 10, Day 13, Day 17, Day 20, Day 24, and Day 27. They are carefully placed to give your body the recovery it needs between the most demanding sessions.

A rest day is not a missed session. It is a required part of the program. The muscles and neural pathways being trained during practice sessions consolidate what they have learned during rest. Skipping a rest day to do an extra session does not make the program more effective. It makes it less effective and increases the risk of fatigue and strain.

On rest days, gentle ordinary walking, stretching, or any light activity you normally do is absolutely fine. What to avoid is the deliberate walking exercises from Chapter Four.

Practicing Safely

Always start with the warm-up from Chapter Three before any session. It takes less than two minutes and it prepares the joints for the walking work ahead.

Walk slowly. More slowly than feels natural. The benefit of Tai Chi walking comes from the deliberate pace, not from covering distance. Moving faster reduces the training effect of every exercise.

Keep the chair or a wall within arm's reach in Weeks One and Two. By Week Three, most people are ready to move a step or two further from their safety support. By Week Four, many people are practicing without the chair nearby at all. Let confidence drive that progression, not a schedule.

If you feel dizzy, sharp pain in a joint, or unusually short of breath, stop. Sit down. Rest. If the feeling does not pass quickly, seek medical advice before continuing.

This program is designed to be done daily on practice days. Missing an occasional session is fine. If you miss three or more consecutive days, return to the beginning of the current week rather than trying to jump to where you left off.

Chapter 1

Why Your Walk Changes After 60

You may have noticed it without naming it: something in the way you walk feels different from ten or fifteen years ago. You are not imagining it. The change is real, it has real causes, and it is not inevitable. This chapter explains what is happening and why the exercises in this book address it specifically.

What Happens to Your Walking After 60

Walking looks simple. You put one foot in front of the other and your body moves forward. But what is actually happening is a sophisticated, continuous process that involves dozens of muscles, hundreds of sensory signals, the balance organs in your inner ear, and the part of your brain that coordinates all of these things in real time. When walking feels effortless, it is because all of these systems are working together without you having to think about them.

After 60, some of those systems begin to change. The changes are gradual, and most people don't notice them until something goes wrong, such as a stumble on a surface they would have crossed without a thought five years earlier. But the changes are real, and they are well understood.

The first change is in muscle strength and reaction time. The muscles of the legs, particularly the ones that stabilize the ankle and control the knee during the single-leg balance phase of every step, become slower to activate and easier to fatigue. Every step involves a brief moment when your entire body weight is balanced over one foot. That moment is managed by muscles working at high speed and precision. When those muscles become less reliable, the step becomes less certain.

The second change is in proprioception, which is the body's ability to sense where it is in space without using its eyes. The soles of the feet and the joints of the ankles are packed with sensory receptors that constantly send information to the brain: how the ground feels, how the weight is distributed, whether the surface is tilting. After 60, the sensitivity of these receptors decreases, and the signals they send become slower and less detailed. The brain gets a fuzzier picture of what is happening under your feet.

The third change is in processing speed. Even if the sensory signals from the feet are reasonably clear, the brain needs time to act on them. A stumble response takes a fraction of a second. As the nervous system ages, that fraction of a second becomes longer. The gap between stumble and corrective response, once fast enough to be invisible, is now just long enough to cause a fall.

None of these changes are dramatic on their own. Together, they add up to a walking pattern that has become slightly less reliable than it used to be. The person who used to walk on autopilot now has to pay a small amount of conscious attention to walking. The walk that felt natural now requires a little more thought. The confidence that was taken for granted has become something that needs to be maintained.

Before naming what this program does about these changes, it is worth being clear about what the word training means in this context. Training does not mean pushing harder. For the nervous system, the most effective stimulus is not high intensity. It is high quality: slow, deliberate, attentive repetition of movements that challenge the specific systems being targeted. Ten minutes of precise, slow, fully attentive walking is more effective at retraining the proprioceptive system than an hour of ordinary walking done on automatic. The number of repetitions matters less than the quality of each one.

There is also a psychological dimension to these physical changes that is worth naming directly. Once a person has stumbled, slipped, or fallen, the experience leaves a trace. The nervous system treats a fall as evidence of danger, and in response it does something that seems helpful but is not: it tenses the muscles, tightens the gait, and shifts more attention toward monitoring the ground. A tense, shortened walk is actually more prone to falling than a relaxed one, because the muscles cannot make the rapid micro-adjustments that balance requires when they are held in a state of constant bracing. The fear of falling can make falling more likely. This is the cycle that this program is designed to break.

It is also worth knowing that the changes in walking after 60 are not the same for everyone. Some people notice them early, in their early sixties, often after a period of illness, reduced activity, or a significant life change. Others do not notice any difference until their mid-seventies. The timing depends on overall activity levels, health history, medication effects, and many other factors. What is consistent is this: the changes are gradual, they are largely reversible with the right training, and they do not wait to be addressed. The earlier deliberate walking training begins, the larger the benefit.

What is important to understand is that these changes are not fixed. The body can be trained to manage them. The muscles can be strengthened. The proprioceptive sensors can be stimulated and maintained. The neural pathways that manage the corrective responses can be made faster and more reliable through specific, deliberate practice. That is exactly what this program provides.

It is also worth understanding that the changes described above are not separate problems happening independently. They interact with each other. Reduced proprioception makes the muscles work harder to compensate, which fatigues them faster. Fatigued muscles respond more slowly. Slower responses increase the risk of a full stumble rather than a caught one. The chain is linked, which means that training any one part of the chain improves the whole. Improved proprioception reduces the compensation demand on the muscles. Less fatigued muscles respond faster. Faster responses improve fall prevention. The program works on multiple parts of the chain simultaneously.

Why Everyday Walk Doesn't Keep You Safe

Many older adults walk regularly. They walk to the shops, around the block, through the garden. They assume that because they walk, their walking is being maintained. In a general sense, this is true. But ordinary walking at an ordinary pace does not challenge the specific systems that falling most depends on.

When you walk at your normal pace on a familiar route, your nervous system uses automatic, well-practiced patterns that require very little active management. The brain is not being asked to solve new balance problems. The muscles are not being pushed to respond faster than usual. The proprioceptive system is being used, but not stretched. The walk is comfortable precisely because it is not asking much.

The problem is that falls rarely happen on familiar routes at a comfortable pace. They happen on unfamiliar ground, at a transition point, in a moment of distraction, or when something unexpected appears underfoot. These are exactly the situations that ordinary comfortable walking does not prepare you for, because ordinary comfortable walking never practices them.

Fall prevention requires practicing the situations that cause falls, in a controlled and safe way. It requires deliberately slowing down so the body has to actively manage each step rather than flowing through it on automatic. It requires practicing weight transfer from one foot to the other with full attention, so the stabilizing muscles are asked to work precisely. It requires practicing direction changes, stops, and starts so the nervous system learns to handle the less predictable moments that real-world walking always contains.

This is why dedicated walking training exists. Not to walk more, but to walk better, and to walk better specifically in the ways that make the difference between a stumble that is caught and a stumble that is not.

Walking training for fall prevention is not about walking more. It is about walking smarter. There is a meaningful difference between covering distance and training balance. A twenty-minute walk on a familiar flat path covers distance and provides cardiovascular benefit. A ten-minute Tai Chi walking session on the same path, with full attention to heel placement, weight transfer, and breath coordination, provides balance training. Both matter. Neither replaces the other. This program addresses the balance training that ordinary walking does not provide and that is most directly related to fall prevention. The two activities are complementary, not interchangeable. Keep your regular walks. Add these ten minutes.

The other problem with relying on ordinary daily walking as a substitute for dedicated practice is that it avoids exactly the surfaces and situations where falls are most likely. People who are worried about their balance instinctively choose smooth, familiar routes and avoid the unpredictable situations that challenge their balance. This is understandable. It is also counterproductive. The balance system improves by encountering managed challenges, not by avoiding all challenges. A program that gradually and safely introduces the more demanding walking situations is exactly what ordinary daily walking cannot provide and what this program does.

Tai Chi Walking Vs. Regular Exercise

Tai Chi walking is not faster or more athletic than ordinary walking. It is slower. Deliberately, specifically slower. That slowness is not a limitation. It is the mechanism.

When you walk slowly enough that each step requires conscious attention, several things happen that do not happen at ordinary walking pace. First, the brain has to actively manage each weight transfer rather than relying on automatic patterns. This activates the motor circuits that handle balance in novel situations, the exact circuits that are responsible for catching stumbles. Second, the proprioceptive system has time to register the full range of sensory information from the feet and ankles before the next step begins. The ground is read more thoroughly. Third, the muscles that stabilize the ankle and knee are asked to hold each position for longer, which builds the endurance and precision they need to function reliably in the uncertain moments.

Tai Chi walking also incorporates specific techniques that ordinary walking does not. The heel-to-toe weight transfer that is central to the Grounded Heel Step exercise teaches the foot to read the ground before loading full weight onto it. The deliberate arm swing of the Arm-Swing Coordination Walk trains the connection between upper and lower body movement that makes the whole walking pattern more stable. The side step exercises train the lateral balance system that is rarely challenged by forward walking and that plays a critical role in catching an unexpected sideways stumble.

The pace of Tai Chi walking also produces a specific biological benefit. Slow, rhythmic movement with coordinated breathing activates the part of the nervous system that calms the body down. Cortisol levels drop. Muscle tension reduces. The person who was walking with braced muscles and a tight grip on their anxiety releases that tension and finds that the walk becomes more fluid. Fluidity is not just more pleasant. It is safer. A tense, rigid walker is more likely to fall than a relaxed, responsive one, because rigidity prevents the automatic micro-adjustments that balance depends on.

None of this requires Tai Chi expertise. The exercises in this book take the core principles of Tai Chi walking, the deliberate pace, the coordinated movement, the attention to weight transfer, and translate them into clear, practical exercises that any older adult can follow without any prior experience.

One more difference that sets Tai Chi walking apart from general exercise is the quality of attention it requires. When you walk while listening to a podcast or talking to a friend, your attention is divided. When you walk with the specific intention of noticing each heel placement, feeling the weight move forward, and timing your breath with your steps, your full attention is on the movement. This quality of focused, deliberate attention is called mindfulness in some contexts, and the research on its effects on balance is clear: people who walk with deliberate attention are steadier and more responsive to unexpected perturbations than people who walk distracted. This program builds that quality of attention from the very first session.

Fall Prevention, Balance, and Confidence

The three goals named in this book's title are not separate objectives that require separate programs. They are the same goal, approached from three directions, and they support each other.

Fall prevention is the most urgent for many people. But fall prevention is not achieved by being more careful or more cautious. It is achieved by having a body that responds faster and more reliably when something unexpected happens underfoot. That response is built through training. The training that builds it is exactly the training that also builds balance and confidence.

Balance is the physical foundation. It is what the walking exercises in this program directly develop. Better balance means the body handles the single-leg moments of each step with more precision. It means the corrective response to a stumble arrives faster. It means the ankle and hip stabilizers are working at the level the situation demands rather than just barely managing. As balance improves, falls become less likely. That is direct, mechanical fall prevention.

Confidence is the outcome that changes daily life the most. A person with good physical balance who is still afraid to walk on uneven ground will avoid it, limit their movement, and gradually lose the capacity they have worked to build. A person with good physical balance and the confidence to use it goes places, stays active, and maintains the physical condition that the confidence depends on. Confidence and physical capacity reinforce each other. The program builds both, and it builds them together rather than separately.

This program builds all three of these goals together rather than treating them as separate targets. The physical exercises build the balance. The graduated confidence comes from successfully completing movements that previously felt uncertain. The fall prevention comes from both. Progress in any one area supports the other two, because they share the same underlying mechanism: a nervous system that has been trained to manage walking more reliably.

By the end of this program, you will have a clearer picture of what has changed and what still needs work. You will have practiced walking in ways that your daily routes do not provide. And you will have a set of exercises you can return to any time your confidence needs refreshing or your balance needs attention. The program has a beginning and an end. The practice it teaches does not.

There is one more thing worth saying about the relationship between these three goals. The person who improves their balance but stays indoors because they don't trust themselves outside has achieved something physically real but practically limited. The person who feels more confident but has not done the work to build the physical foundation for that confidence is relying on a feeling rather than a capacity. This program builds both together, in proportion, with the physical training always a little ahead of where the confidence needs to go, so that when the confidence arrives, it is supported by something real.

Chapter 2

The Science Behind Safer Steps

You do not need to understand the science to benefit from this program. But knowing why each piece works will help you pay attention in the right places during practice and get more from every session.

How Your Balance System Works

Your balance system is not one thing. It is three systems working together, and it is as good as the weakest of the three.

The first system is your vision. Your eyes continuously give your brain information about where your body is in relation to the world around it. When you look at a fixed point on the wall, your brain uses that information to keep you upright. When the surface under your feet changes or when your footing is uncertain, most people instinctively look down at their feet. This is a natural response, but it is not always helpful. Watching your feet as you walk reduces the information your eyes can give your brain about what is coming next, and it shifts your center of gravity forward, which actually makes falling slightly more likely.

The second system is your vestibular system, which is located in your inner ear. The inner ear contains fluid-filled canals and tiny sensory hairs that detect the direction and speed of head movement. When your head tilts, the fluid moves, the hairs respond, and your brain receives information about which way is up and how fast you are moving. The vestibular system is particularly important during the head movements that walking involves, and it works closely with the visual system to keep the picture of the world stable even when the head is moving.

The third system is proprioception. This is the body's internal sense of where it is in space. The joints, muscles, and especially the soles of the feet are packed with sensory receptors that continuously monitor position, pressure, and movement. When your weight shifts forward over the front foot, proprioceptive signals from the ankle and foot tell the brain exactly what is happening, before the eyes or inner ear can register it. Proprioception is your fastest and most detailed balance information source.

After 60, all three systems become somewhat less reliable, but proprioception declines the fastest. The sensory receptors in the feet become less sensitive. The ankles send slower and less precise signals to the brain. The brain's ability to integrate proprioceptive information with visual and vestibular information takes slightly longer. The result is a balance system that is still functional but operating with less precision and less speed than it once had.

This is why falls often happen in situations that seem straightforward: stepping off a curb that was slightly higher than expected, crossing the threshold between two types of flooring, walking on a surface that looks even but isn't. In each of these cases, the problem is not that the person lacked the strength or awareness to manage the situation. It is that the information arrived too slowly for the response to catch the stumble in time. Proprioceptive training addresses this directly: it gives the receptors more practice, the pathways more use, and the brain a more reliable and faster stream of information to act on.

The walking exercises in this program are specifically designed to train proprioception. Every exercise that asks you to slow down and feel each step is giving the sensory receptors in your feet more time to register the surface. Every exercise that asks you to transfer weight deliberately from one foot to the other is asking the ankle proprioceptors to work precisely. Over four weeks of daily deliberate practice, these receptors become more responsive, and the signals they send become faster and more reliable.

You can experience the difference between well-trained and under-trained proprioception with a simple test. Stand on one foot on a smooth, flat floor and count how long you can balance without grabbing for support. Now try the same thing on a slightly uneven surface, such as a folded towel. The difficulty increase on the uneven surface reflects how much your balance currently depends on the visual system as a backup for insufficient proprioceptive information. As this program progresses, the uneven-surface balance will improve more than the flat-surface balance, because the proprioceptive training is specifically addressing the receptors that the variable surface activates.

Role of Muscle Memory in Every Step You Take

Muscle memory is not actually stored in the muscles. It is stored in the brain, in networks of neural pathways that have been strengthened through repetition until the movement they represent can be performed without conscious thought. When you learned to ride a bike or to write your name, you were building muscle memory. Once it is built, the movement can be recalled without effort and without thinking.

Walking is built on muscle memory. The basic pattern of putting one foot in front of the other is so deeply embedded in the nervous system by adulthood that it requires almost no conscious attention. This is why you can walk and hold a conversation at the same time without either activity suffering. The walking is handled by automatic neural programs while the conscious mind handles the conversation.

The problem is that automatic programs do not update themselves in response to changing conditions. If the muscles and sensory systems that the automatic walking program depends on become less reliable, the program still runs. It just runs on less reliable hardware. The person whose ankle proprioception has declined does not automatically develop a new walking pattern to compensate. They walk the same way, with the same automatic program, but the results are less reliable than they used to be.

Deliberate practice is how you update the program. When you walk slowly enough that each step requires conscious attention, you are no longer using the automatic program. You are working in the deliberate learning mode of the nervous system. In this mode, new neural pathways can be built and strengthened. Old pathways that have become sluggish can be retrained. The brain can learn to manage weight transfer more precisely, to respond faster to unexpected surface changes, and to use the available proprioceptive information more efficiently.

This is why the slow pace of Tai Chi walking is not a compromise. It is the mechanism. Fast automatic walking uses and reinforces the existing automatic program. Slow deliberate walking builds and strengthens a better one.

One practical insight from the research on motor learning is that blocked practice, repeating the same movement many times in a row, is less effective for skill retention than variable practice, mixing different but related movements within the same session. This is why the

28-day program in this book introduces new exercises progressively and then keeps earlier exercises in the rotation rather than dropping them. The brain learns better when it has to apply similar skills in slightly different contexts. Each week adds new exercises rather than replacing old ones, which keeps the nervous system adapting throughout the program.

The exercises in this program are sequenced to make this rebuilding as effective as possible. The simplest exercises come first. As the neural pathways for those exercises strengthen, the next exercises introduce slightly greater challenges. Each exercise adds something the previous one did not demand: a slightly wider step, a direction change, a moment of single-leg balance, an obstacle to step over. By the time the more complex exercises appear in Weeks Three and Four, the nervous system has been prepared for them by the earlier work. The progression is deliberate, and it is based on how neural adaptation actually works.

How Mindful Walking Retrains the Nervous System

The nervous system learns by repetition. A movement that is practiced hundreds of times becomes encoded in neural pathways that are strong, fast, and reliable. A movement that is practiced occasionally, or under conditions of stress and distraction, produces weaker, less reliable pathways. The quality of the repetition matters as much as the number.

High-quality repetition means performing the movement with full attention, at a pace that allows the nervous system to process all the relevant sensory information, and without the distraction of competing demands. This is exactly the condition that the exercises in this program create. Each exercise is short. The pace is slow. The attention is directed at specific aspects of the movement: the feel of the heel on the floor, the moment of weight transfer, the steadiness of the leading step.

When walking is practiced in this way, the neural pathways that manage balance during walking become stronger and more precise. The brain learns to use the proprioceptive information from the feet more efficiently. The automatic corrective responses that prevent stumbles become faster. The muscles that stabilize each step develop better coordination and endurance.

The breathing that accompanies Tai Chi walking adds another layer. Slow, deliberate breathing during exercise activates the parasympathetic nervous system, which reduces muscle tension and lowers the stress response. A person practicing Tai Chi walking is not just training their balance. They are simultaneously reducing the cortisol-driven tension that makes the muscles less responsive and the nervous system less accurate. The calm that Tai Chi walking produces is not separate from the balance training. It is part of it.

There is also a practical reason why the calming effect matters beyond the session itself. People who have had a fall or a serious scare often carry an ambient level of tension into every subsequent walk. That tension, the slight bracing against a fall that might happen, actually disrupts the fluid, responsive movement that prevents falls. Breaking this cycle requires two things: better physical capacity and the experience of walking calmly. The deliberate breathing of Tai Chi walking provides both in the same session, every session.

Findings on Tai Chi and Fall Prevention

Tai Chi is one of the most researched exercise interventions for fall prevention in older adults. The findings are consistent across many studies conducted over many years and in many countries. Here are the main things the research has established, stated in plain terms.

First, regular Tai Chi practice reduces the number of falls in older adults. Studies have found reductions in fall rate ranging from around 20 percent to over 40 percent compared to control groups, with the greatest benefits seen in people who practice consistently for at least 12 weeks. The effects are not subtle. They are meaningful and measurable.

Second, the balance improvements from Tai Chi are specific to the kinds of balance challenges that cause real-world falls. It is not just that participants score better on laboratory balance tests. They also show faster corrective responses to unexpected perturbations, better performance on uneven surfaces, and reduced fear of falling in daily situations. These are the outcomes that actually prevent falls in the places where falls happen.

Third, the cognitive component matters. Tai Chi requires the kind of sustained, sequential attention that other forms of walking exercise do not. Studies have found that this cognitive engagement, learning and maintaining the forms, produces improvements in reaction time, attention, and processing speed that transfer to non-exercise situations. The person who practices Tai Chi walking becomes more alert in general, which makes their responses to unexpected situations faster and more accurate.

Fourth, it is never too late to benefit. Studies have found significant improvements in balance and fall risk in adults in their 70s and 80s who had no prior Tai Chi experience. The nervous system retains the ability to learn and adapt throughout life. The training works at every age.

This program draws directly on these findings. The exercises are designed to provide exactly the kind of deliberate, slow, attention-requiring walking practice that the research shows to be effective. The 28-day structure is long enough to produce real neurological adaptation and short enough to be a realistic commitment. The progress checks allow you to see your own improvements against your own baseline, which is more meaningful than any population average.

Chapter 3

Setting Yourself Up for Success

Getting the setup right takes five minutes. It makes every session safer and more effective. This chapter walks through everything you need to check, prepare, and know before Day 1 begins.

Check In With Your Body Before Each Session

Every session in this program starts the same way: with a quick check of how the body feels today. This is not a medical assessment. It is two minutes of honest attention to the areas that will be doing the most work.

The joints most involved in walking are the ankles, knees, and hips. Before each session, notice each of these in turn. Rotate each ankle gently in both directions. Bend and straighten each knee slowly. Shift your weight from one hip to the other. You are looking for two things: normal morning stiffness that eases with movement, and something more specific that needs attention.

Normal morning stiffness is the aching, creaky sensation that most people over 60 feel for the first ten or twenty minutes after getting up. It eases as the joints warm up and the synovial fluid circulates. It is not a reason to skip the session. In fact, the walking exercises in this program are specifically designed to address it. Starting with the warm-up routine described later in this chapter will resolve most of this stiffness before the main session begins.

A specific signal, sharp pain in one location, a joint that feels swollen or significantly hotter than usual, or pain that does not ease at all with gentle movement, is a different matter. If any of these are present, take the day as a rest day and reassess the following morning. If a specific joint has been consistently painful or swollen for three or more days, speak with your doctor before continuing the program.

Balance is the other pre-session check. Stand near a wall or the back of a chair for a moment and notice whether your balance feels usual today or notably less steady than normal. Some days are simply more unsteady than others, for reasons that have nothing to do with the program: a disrupted night's sleep, minor illness, a change in medication. On an unsteady day, keep the chair or wall closer than usual throughout the session and use the low-energy session option from the Chapter Five entry for that day.

> **SAFETY NOTE:**
> If you feel dizzy on waking, do the pre-session check seated rather than standing. Dizziness on waking that does not resolve within a few minutes is worth reporting to your doctor, particularly if it is a new symptom.

What to Wear, Where to Walk, and What to Avoid

What to Wear

Footwear.

The right shoe for this program is flat, well-fitting, and non-slip. The sole should be firm enough to provide stability but not so thick that it reduces the sensation of the ground underfoot. Sensation matters: the proprioceptive receptors in the soles of the feet read the surface through the shoe, and a very thick cushioned sole muffles that reading. Canvas walking shoes, leather-soled flat shoes, or low-profile sports shoes all work well. Sandals, backless shoes, slip-on shoes that do not fit snugly, and shoes with worn or uneven soles are all unsuitable for this program.

If you wear orthotics, wear them throughout every session. They are part of the mechanical system that the exercises are training. Leaving them out during practice and wearing them the rest of the time creates an inconsistency that reduces the quality of the proprioceptive training.

Laces should be tied securely before every session. A loose lace is a trip hazard that the most sophisticated balance training cannot overcome.

Clothing.

Wear clothing that allows free movement through the hips, knees, and arms. Tight trousers or a skirt that restricts leg movement will limit the stride length and the side-stepping range of certain exercises. Layers are better than a single heavy garment, particularly for outdoor sessions, because they allow you to adjust to changing temperature without having to stop the session.

Where to walk.

For Weeks One and Two, indoor practice on a clear, flat, non-slip floor is the recommended starting point. A hallway, a long clear room, or a garage floor all work. The path should be at least ten feet long without requiring a turn, though longer is better for the exercises that involve continuous walking. Remove rugs, electrical cables, and any object at floor level that is not immediately obvious. The pre-session environment check takes thirty seconds and eliminates the most common indoor trip hazards.

From Week Three onward, outdoor walking on a flat, familiar pavement or path becomes appropriate. Begin with a route you know well, in good lighting, on a surface you trust. Introduce new or more challenging outdoor environments gradually, following the progression described in Chapter Seven.

What to avoid.

Avoid thick-pile carpet for the first two weeks. It makes the heel-first landing mechanics harder to feel and execute, and it reduces the ground-reading sensation that the early exercises depend on. Avoid wet or recently polished floors. Avoid walking in socks without shoes on smooth surfaces. Avoid sessions when you are significantly fatigued, unwell, or have recently taken any medication that lists dizziness as a side effect.

> **NOTE:**
> If outdoor practice is not available due to weather or mobility constraints, all twelve exercises in this program can be done indoors throughout the full 28 days. The indoor practice is not a reduced version. It is a complete version.

The Warm-Up Routine

The warm-up takes two to three minutes and is done before every session, without exception. It serves two purposes: it circulates synovial fluid through the walking joints before they are asked to bear full body weight under the training exercises, and it brings attention into the body before the session begins. Both purposes matter.

Do the warm-up standing beside the chair, with one hand available to touch it if needed. Move through the following sequence slowly and without forcing any joint into a range that feels sharp.

Ankle Circles

Starting Position: Standing beside the chair, weight on the left foot, right foot raised slightly.

1. Shift weight to the left foot. Lift the right foot just off the floor.

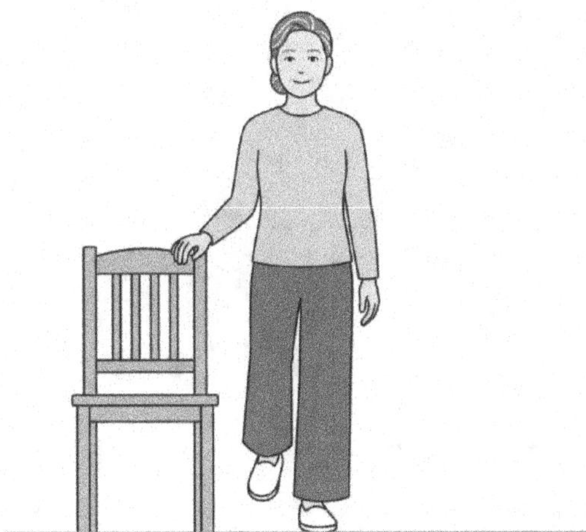

2. Rotate the ankle slowly in a circle, five times clockwise, five times counterclockwise.

3. Lower the right foot. Shift weight to the right foot.

4. Lift the left foot and repeat ankle rotation.

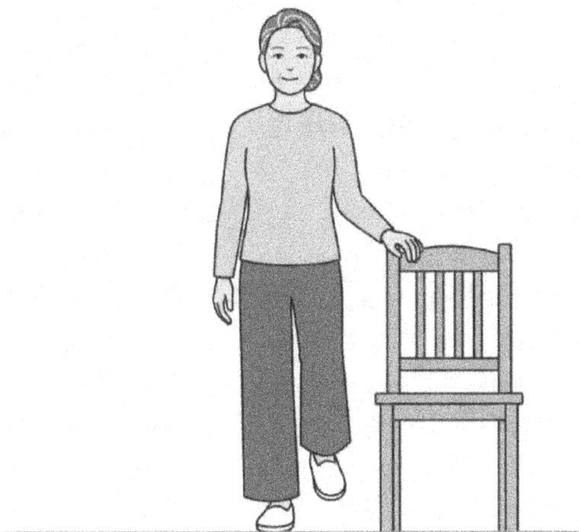

FEEL IT: A gentle mobilization through the ankle joint, particularly in the areas that feel stiffest. The movement should ease the stiffness, not increase it.

Knee Bends

Starting Position: Standing behind the chair, both hands resting lightly on the chair back. Feet hip-width apart, flat on the floor.

1. Hold the chair back lightly for balance.
2. Bend both knees slowly into a shallow squat, roughly a quarter of the way down. Keep the heels flat on the floor.

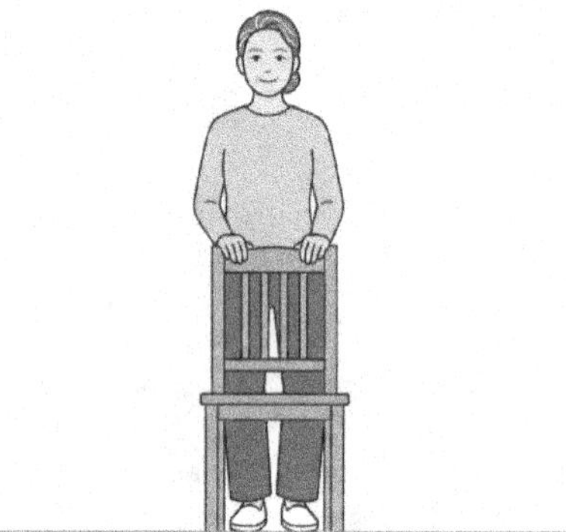

3. Hold for two counts at the bottom.
4. Straighten slowly back to standing.
5. Repeat five times. Do not go deeper than is comfortable.

FEEL IT: A warm engagement in the front of the thighs and a gentle opening sensation in the knee joint as the fluid distributes.

> **SAFETY NOTE:**
> Do not push the knee bend deeper than is comfortable. A very shallow bend is fine. The purpose is joint mobilization, not strength training.

Hip Circles

Starting Position: Standing with feet shoulder-width apart, both hands resting lightly on hips. Weight centered.

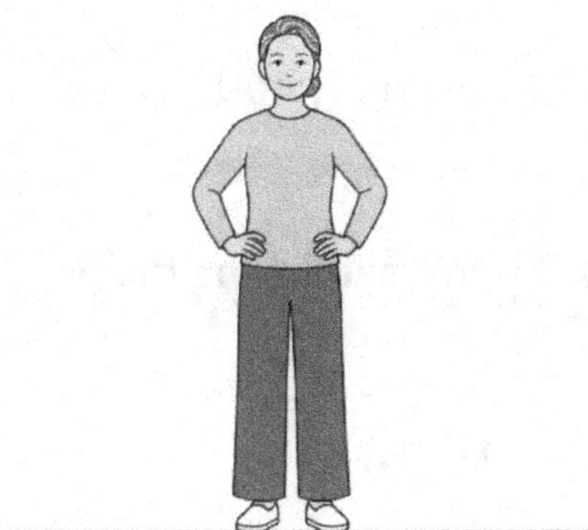

1. Keep the feet still and the upper body relatively upright.

2. Move the pelvis slowly in a horizontal circle: forward, right, back, left, and forward again.

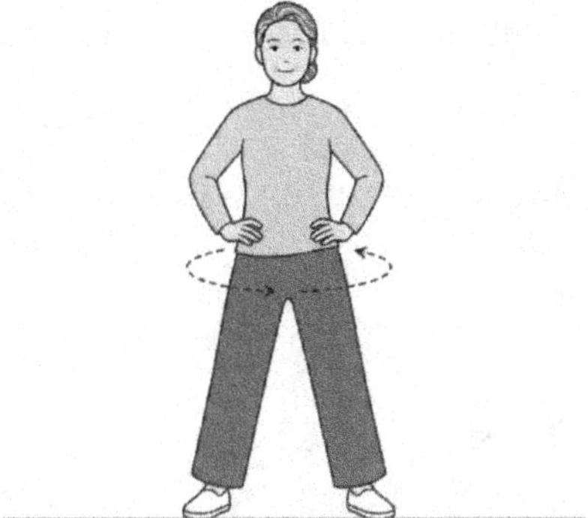

3. Complete five circles in one direction.

4. Reverse for five circles in the other direction.

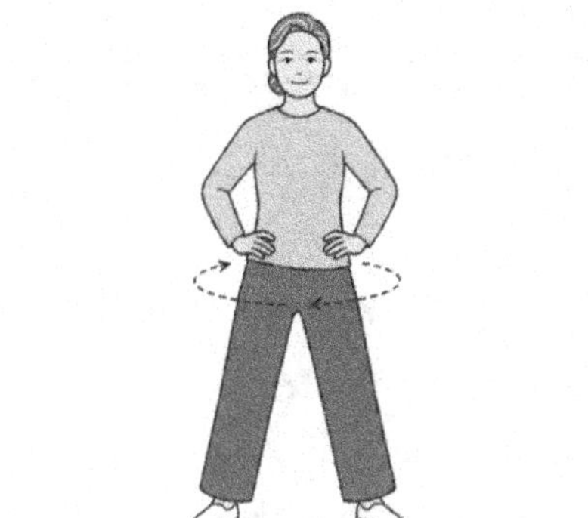

FEEL IT: A loosening sensation through the hip joints and the lower back as the circular movement works the joint through a range that ordinary standing does not provide.

Calf Raises

Starting Position: Standing behind the chair, both hands on the chair back. Feet hip-width apart.

1. Rise slowly onto the balls of both feet, lifting the heels off the floor.
2. Hold at the top for one count.
3. Lower the heels slowly back to the floor.
4. Repeat eight times. Move slowly up and slowly down on every repetition.

FEEL IT: A clear engagement in the calf muscles and a stretching sensation through the Achilles tendon on the way back down.

After completing the four warm-up movements, stand still for a moment and notice how the joints feel compared to before the warm-up. Most people feel a noticeable difference in ankle and knee mobility after even this brief sequence. That difference is synovial fluid reaching the cartilage surfaces that the walking exercises will use. The warm-up is doing real work in those two to three minutes.

Your Day One Walking Baseline

These three tests are done on the same day as the Chapter Three warm-up, before Day 1 of the program. They take about five minutes altogether. Write the results down and keep them somewhere accessible, because the progress checks at the end of each week in Chapter Five will return to them.

The purpose is not to score yourself. There are no good or bad results. The purpose is to have a specific, honest starting point so that the Day 28 results are a genuine comparison rather than a vague impression.

> **Baseline Test 1: Single-Leg Balance Hold**
> Stand beside the chair with one hand available to touch it.
> Shift your weight onto the right foot. Lift the left foot just a few centimeters off the floor.
> Release the chair and count how many seconds you can hold the position before needing to touch the chair or put the left foot down.
> Write down the number. Repeat on the other side.
> Record both: Right side: seconds. Left side: seconds.

Most adults over 60 manage between 5 and 20 seconds per side on this test at the start of the program. There is no minimum required to begin. Whatever your number, it will improve.

Baseline Test 2: Heel-to-Toe Walk (10 Steps)
Stand at one end of a clear walking path.
Walk forward placing each foot so the heel touches directly in front of the previous toe, as if walking along a narrow line.
Count how many steps you complete before needing to step sideways to recover balance.
Write down the number. If you complete all 10 without breaking, write 10.
Record: Number of heel-to-toe steps completed before stepping out:

This test measures narrow-line balance directly. Most people starting this program manage between 3 and 7 steps before needing to widen their base. Again, there is no minimum. The number will change.

Baseline Test 3: Comfortable Walking Pace Self-Rating
Take an ordinary short walk of about 20 steps at your usual comfortable pace, indoors.
Rate your confidence on a scale of 1 to 5: 1 is very unsteady and worried, 5 is completely confident with no concerns.
Write down your rating.
Record: Confidence rating (1-5):

This third baseline is the most subjective, but it is often the most meaningful by Day 28. Changes in walking confidence are real changes even when balance test numbers are slow to move.

NOTE:
Keep your three baseline numbers someplace you can easily come back to or place just within this page as a bookmark. The Day 28 progress check will ask for them by name.

With the warm-up practiced and the three baselines recorded, you are ready for Day 1. Chapter Four describes all twelve exercises before you need to use them. Read through it now, even if only briefly, so that the exercises in Chapter Five are not completely new when they first appear.

Chapter 4

The Twelve Tai Chi Walking Exercises

These are the twelve exercises that make up the 28-day program. Read through all of them before Day 1. You don't need to memorize them, but seeing each one first means you won't be learning a new movement cold in the middle of a session.

How to Read Each Exercise Block

Every exercise in this chapter is laid out the same way. First, the name and a plain-English description of what the exercise is for. Then two or three images showing the starting position and the key movement. Then numbered steps, starting at 1 for every exercise. After the steps, three cue labels: FEEL IT tells you what correct movement should feel like in your body. SAFETY TIP points out the single most important thing to watch out for. CONFIDENCE NOTE explains how this exercise connects to safer, more confident real-world walking. Finally, a Modification box explains how to make the exercise easier if needed.

Walk in flat, non-slip shoes. Keep a sturdy chair or a wall within arm's reach during Weeks One and Two. Move at a pace that feels deliberately slow, slower than your natural walking speed. If an exercise feels too easy at that pace, slow down further rather than adding speed. The benefit comes from the pace and the attention, not from covering distance.

Exercise 1: Grounded Heel Step

Teaches you to land on your heel first and feel the ground before your full weight follows. This is the foundation of safe walking and the single most important thing you can train for fall prevention.

Steps:

1. Stand with your feet together at the start of a clear walking path. Look straight ahead.

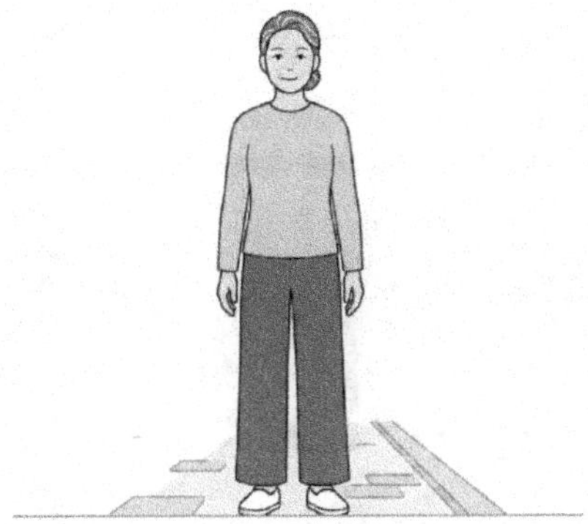

2. Lift your right foot slowly and step forward.

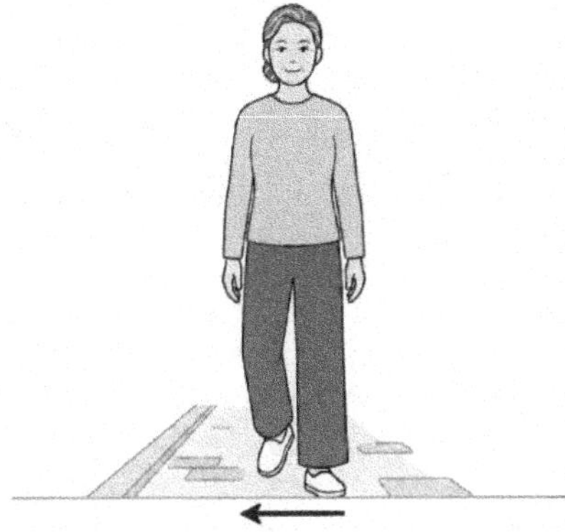

3. Let the heel touch down first. Pause for one count.

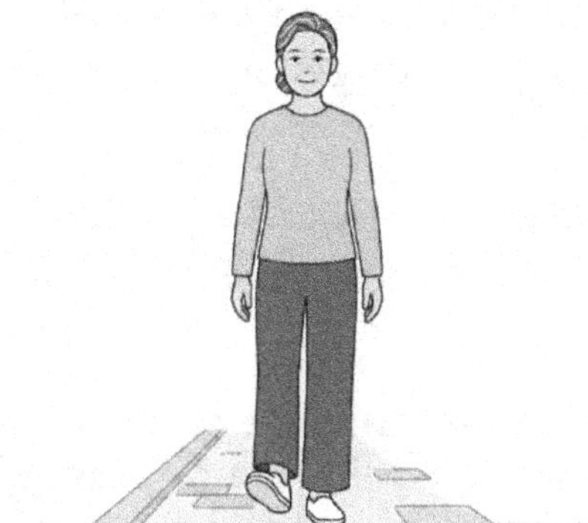

4. Roll your weight forward through the foot, from heel to ball to toe.

5. As your weight moves forward, let the left heel lift naturally.

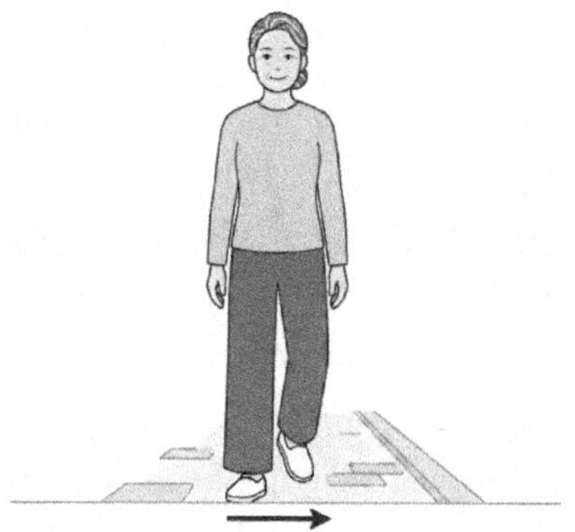

6. Bring the left foot forward the same way: heel first, pause, roll.

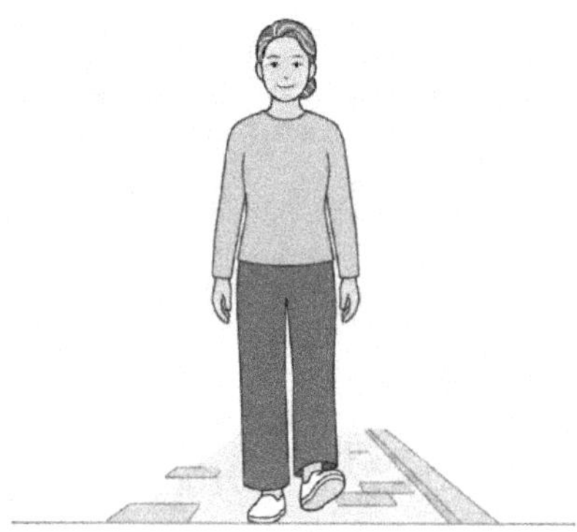

7. Continue for the length of your walking path. Turn carefully and return.

FEEL IT: A clear, deliberate contact between your heel and the floor before your weight transfers. Each step should feel like you are reading the ground before trusting it.

SAFETY TIP: Do not look down at your feet while walking. Keep your eyes forward. The feet will find the ground without you watching them.

CONFIDENCE NOTE: This exercise trains the exact habit that prevents most stumble-related falls: testing the surface before loading your full weight onto it.

> **MODIFICATION:**
> If the heel-first landing is uncomfortable, reduce the step length until it feels manageable. A smaller step is a better step.

Exercise 2: Slow-Motion Forward Walk

Slows the natural walking pace to a deliberate, controlled speed that gives your balance system time to manage each step fully. This is the core speed for all exercises in Weeks One and Two.

Steps:

1. Start at one end of your walking path. Feet together.

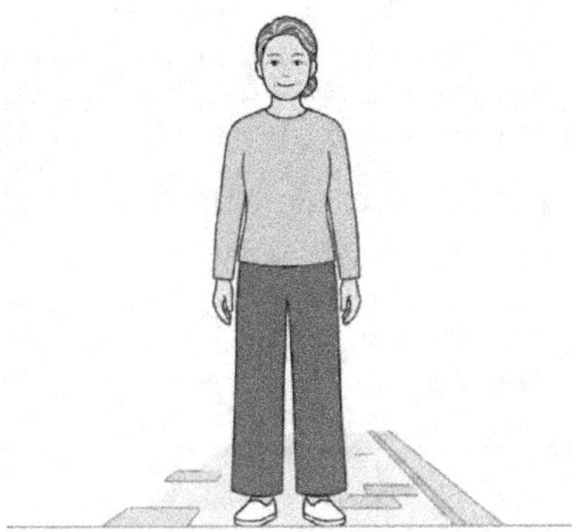

2. Begin walking forward using the Grounded Heel Step from Exercise 1.

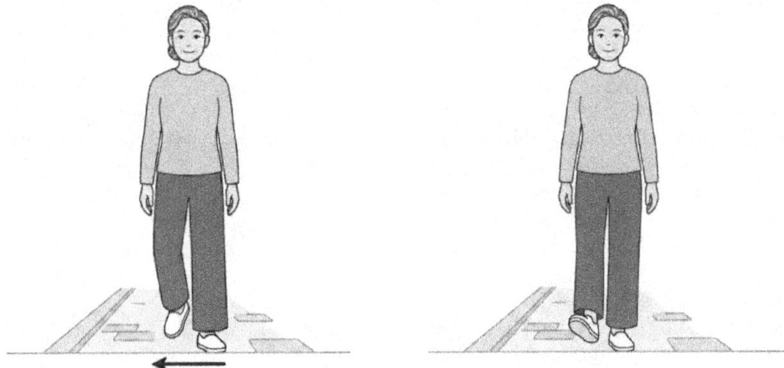

3. Slow your pace to roughly half your normal walking speed. Count one-two in your head with each step if it helps.

4. Let your arms swing gently opposite to your legs: left arm forward as right foot steps, right arm forward as left foot steps.

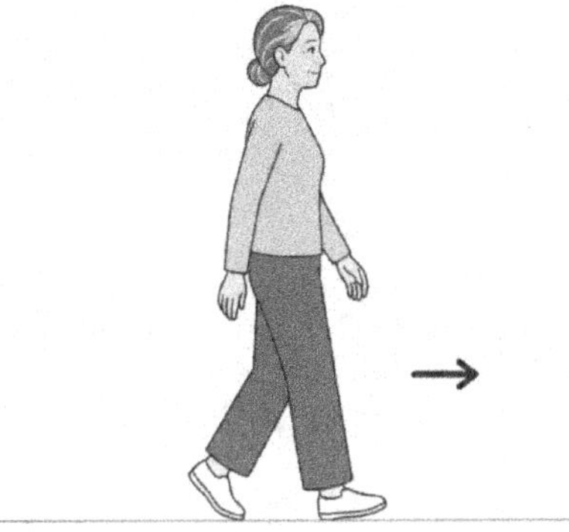

5. Breathe slowly. Inhale for two steps, exhale for two steps.

6. Walk to the end of the path, pause, turn slowly, and return.

7. Complete two full lengths at this pace.

FEEL IT: A quiet, grounded sensation with each step. Your body is in control of the movement rather than flowing through it automatically.

SAFETY TIP: If slowing down makes you feel unsteady, keep a wall or chair within easy reach for the first few sessions.

CONFIDENCE NOTE: Slow, deliberate walking in practice makes your balance system more reliable at all speeds, including your normal everyday pace.

> **MODIFICATION:**
> Walk alongside a wall, close enough to touch it with your fingertips if needed. As confidence grows, move a step further from the wall each session.

Exercise 3: Step and Pause

Adds a deliberate stopping point in the middle of each step to build single-leg balance and retrain the brain to manage weight transfer carefully.

Steps:

1. Begin walking forward at the slow pace from Exercise 2.

2. As your left foot lifts to step forward, pause with it just off the floor for one count.

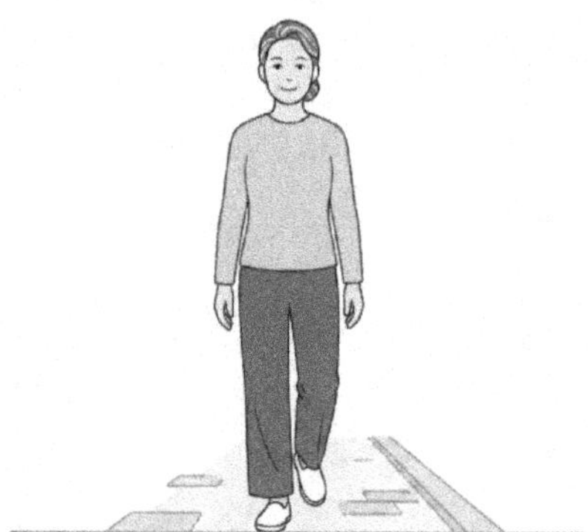

3. Hold the balance on your right foot for that moment.

4. Place the left heel down. Transfer your weight.

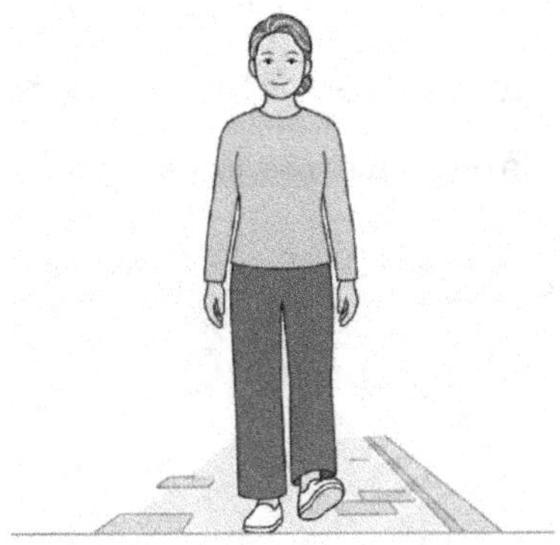

5. As your right foot lifts, pause it off the floor for one count.

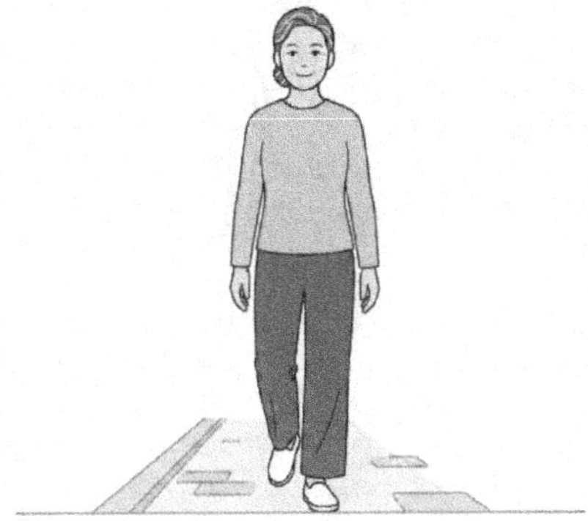

6. Continue: lift, pause, place. One pause on every step.

FEEL IT: A brief moment of single-leg balance with each step. Your ankle will make small adjustments during the pause. This is correct.

SAFETY TIP: Do not lock the standing knee. Keep a slight bend in it throughout. A locked knee makes balance harder, not easier.

CONFIDENCE NOTE: Building this brief pause retrains the automatic stumble response. Your leg learns to stay steady in the single-leg moments that cause most falls.

MODIFICATION:
Reduce the pause to a half-count if a full pause feels too demanding. Build toward a full one-count pause over the first week.

Exercise 4: Toe-Lift Walk

Strengthens the shin muscles and improves foot clearance with every step, reducing the risk of catching a toe on a threshold or an uneven surface.

Steps:

1. Stand at the start of your walking path.

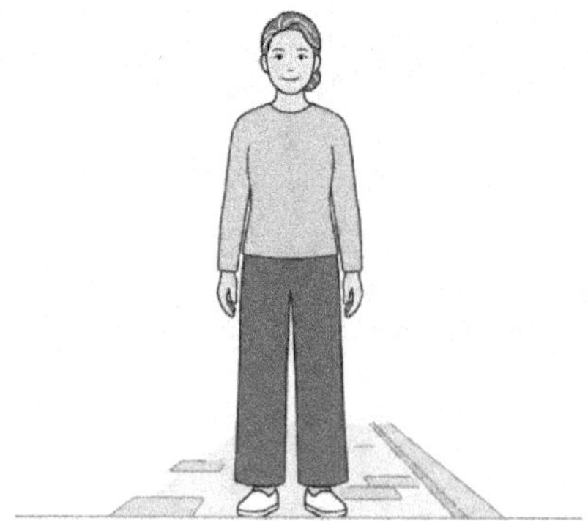

2. As you step forward with each foot, lift the toes up toward the shin as the foot swings through.

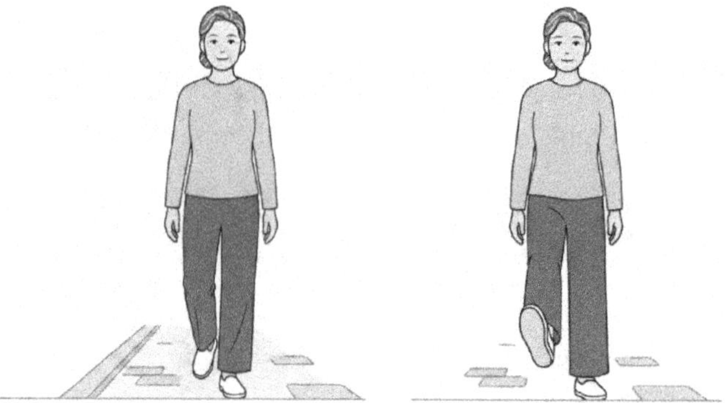

3. Land on the heel with toes still raised.

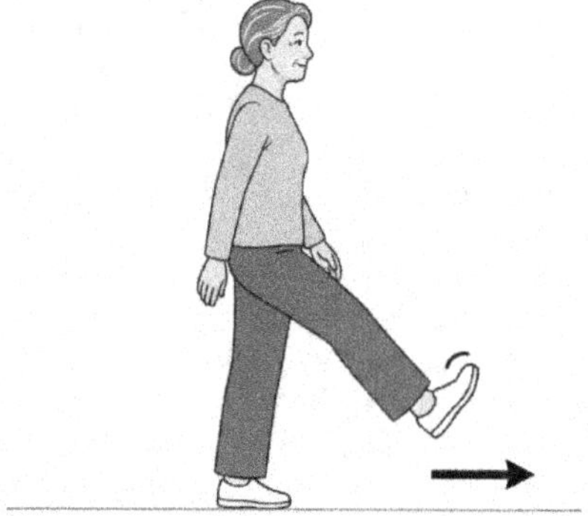

4. Lower the toes slowly as the weight rolls through.

5. Repeat on every step for the length of the path.

6. Keep your pace slow. The toe lift takes more effort than normal walking.

FEEL IT: A mild pulling sensation in the shin muscles as the toes lift. This is the muscle doing its job.

SAFETY TIP: Toe-lift walking is tiring for the shin muscles early on. Stop before fatigue causes you to drag the foot. Better to do less with good form.

CONFIDENCE NOTE: Most trips and stumbles happen because the foot doesn't clear the ground fully. This exercise directly addresses that by strengthening toe lift on every step.

> **MODIFICATION:**
> Raise the toes just slightly if a full lift is uncomfortable. Any deliberate toe lift is more than the foot usually gets.

Exercise 5: Wide-Base Side Step

Trains lateral balance by stepping sideways, which challenges the hip stabilizers that ordinary forward walking rarely tests.

Steps:

1. Stand with feet shoulder-width apart. Face a clear open space to your right.

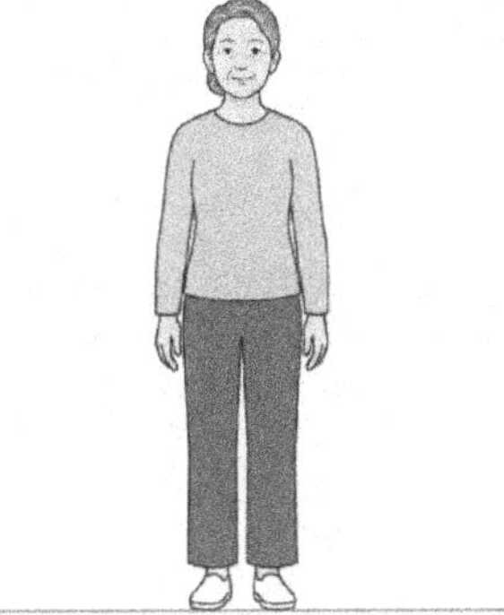

2. Step the right foot out one step to the right.

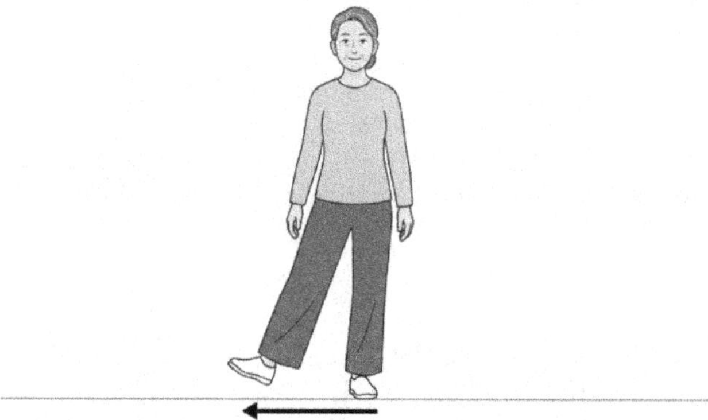

3. Shift your weight fully onto the right foot.

4. Bring the left foot in to meet the right foot. Pause.

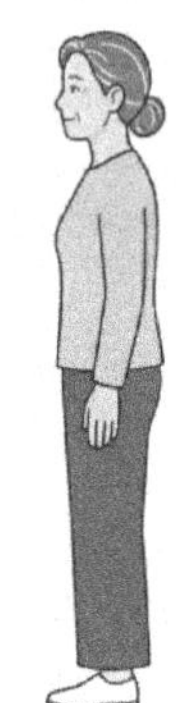

5. Repeat: right step out, weight shift, left foot closes.

6. Complete eight steps to the right.

7. Reverse: step the left foot out to the left, weight shift, right foot closes.

8. Complete eight steps to the left.

FEEL IT: A clear engagement in the outer hip as each step bears full weight. This is the hip stabilizer working.

SAFETY TIP: Keep both feet pointing forward throughout. Do not let the stepping foot turn out as it reaches to the side.

CONFIDENCE NOTE: The side-step muscles are the first ones to respond when you lose balance to the side. Strengthening them reduces the risk of a sideways fall.

Exercise 6: Arm-Swing Coordination Walk

Restores the natural arm-leg coordination of walking, which improves balance and reduces the stiff, shortened stride common in people who walk with caution.

Steps:

1. Begin the Slow-Motion Forward Walk from Exercise 2.

2. As your left foot steps forward, swing your right arm forward at the same time.

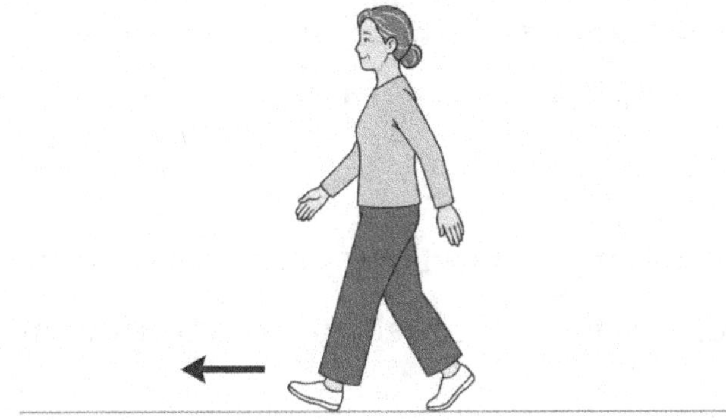

3. As your right foot steps forward, swing your left arm forward.

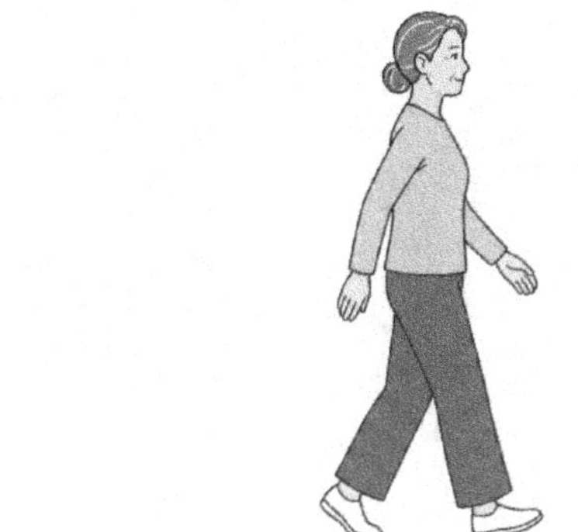

4. Keep the swing relaxed. The arm should move from the shoulder, not just the elbow.

5. Exaggerate the swing slightly more than your natural walk. This is deliberate training.

6. Walk two full lengths of your path.

FEEL IT: A natural, flowing rhythm between the arms and legs. When the coordination is right, the walk should feel slightly easier, not harder.

SAFETY TIP: Do not swing the arms so wide that you lose balance. A moderate, relaxed swing is the goal.

CONFIDENCE NOTE: Arm-swing coordinates the whole body in walking. People who walk with reduced arm movement tend to shuffle, which increases fall risk. This exercise reverses that.

> **MODIFICATION:**
> If coordinating arms and legs feels too demanding at first, walk with arms swinging freely for one session before adding the coordination requirement.

Exercise 7: Heel-to-Toe Precision Walk

Trains narrow-line balance by walking a straight line with each step placed heel directly in front of the previous toe, like walking along a tightrope.

Steps:

1. Stand at the start of a straight line on the floor, or imagine one.
2. Place your right foot forward so the heel touches directly in front of the left toes.

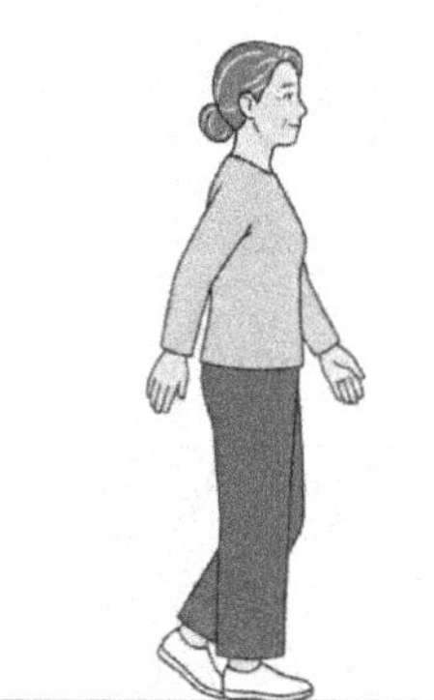

3. Shift your weight fully onto the right foot.
4. Place your left foot forward so its heel touches in front of the right toes.

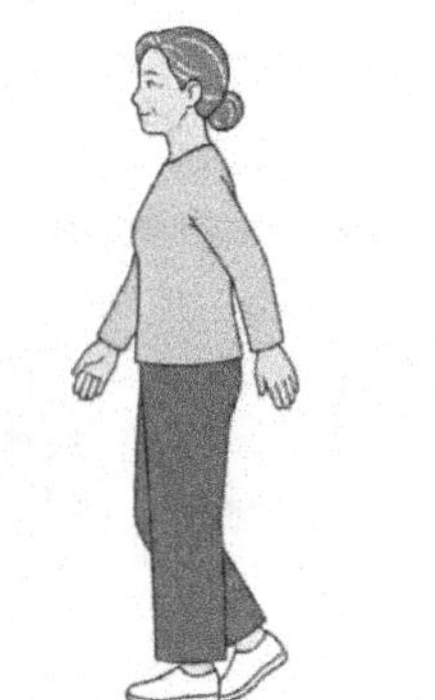

5. Continue for ten steps. Walk slowly. Use a wall or chair back for light fingertip support if needed.

6. Pause at the end. Return along the same line.

FEEL IT: A narrow, focused sensation under each foot. Small ankle movements are normal. This is your balance system working at the fine level.

SAFETY TIP: This is the most balance-demanding exercise in Weeks Three and Four. Always have a chair or wall within easy reach.

CONFIDENCE NOTE: Crowded spaces, narrow aisles, and uneven pavements all require narrow-line balance. This exercise directly builds the skill you need for those situations.

> **MODIFICATION:**
> Place the foot slightly to the side of the line rather than exactly in front if heel-to-toe is too narrow. Narrow the placement gradually over the program.

Exercise 8: Figure-Eight Walking Path

Practices direction changes and gentle curves within a small space, training the balance adjustments needed for turning while walking.

Steps:

1. Place two objects on the floor about four feet apart as turning markers. Shoes, books, or paper plates all work.

2. Begin at one marker and walk forward to the second.

3. Walk around the second marker in a gentle curve, keeping the marker to your right.

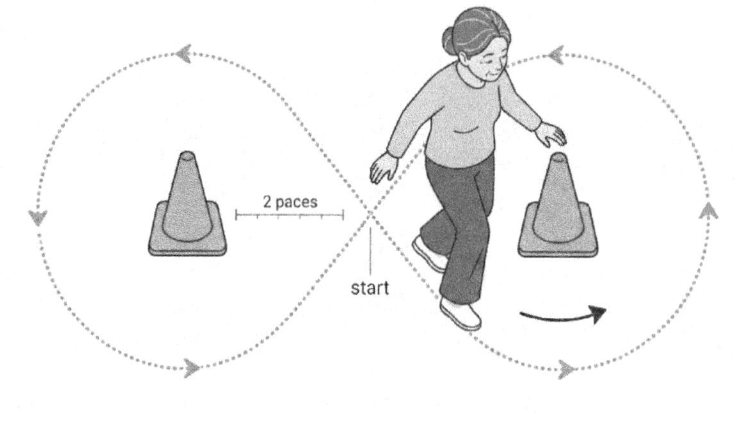

4. Walk back to the first marker and curve around it, keeping it to your right.

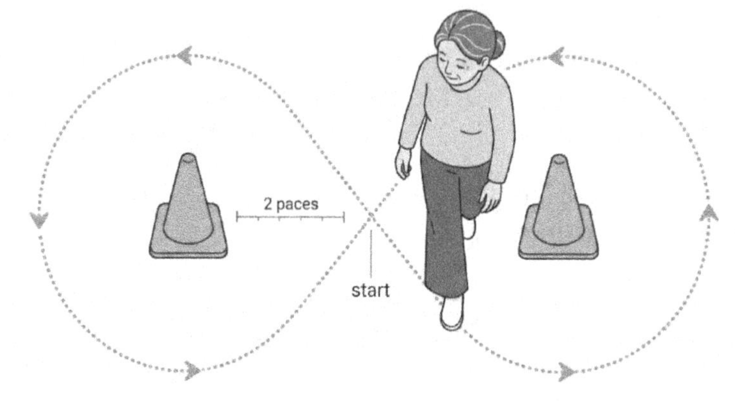

5. Continue the figure-eight pattern: two loops in one direction.

6. Reverse: walk the figure-eight so each marker is to your left.

7. Complete two loops in each direction.

FEEL IT: A slight shift in balance as you enter each curve. Your outer foot will take slightly more weight. Let that happen rather than resisting it.

SAFETY TIP: Take the curves slowly and widely. A sharp turn is harder to balance than a gentle arc.

CONFIDENCE NOTE: Turning while walking is one of the highest-risk moments for falls. Practicing gentle curves in a controlled space makes real-world turns much safer.

Exercise 9: Backward Step and Hold

Builds backward-step confidence and hip extension strength, which are needed for stepping

back away from hazards and recovering from a forward stumble.

Steps:

1. Stand with a clear space behind you. Check the area is free of obstacles before starting.

2. Step your right foot backward one step, landing lightly on the ball of the foot. Arms
    slightly forward for counterbalance

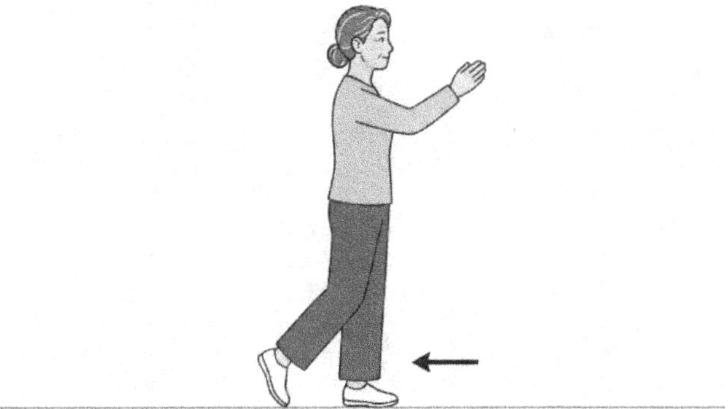

3. Shift your weight back onto the right foot. Pause for one count.

4. Step the left foot back to meet the right foot. Stand still for one count.

5. Continue: right step back, pause, left step back, pause.

6. Complete six backward steps.

7. Walk forward back to the start using Exercise 1.

FEEL IT: A stretch through the front of the hip as the stepping leg reaches backward. This
is the hip flexor lengthening.

SAFETY TIP: Always check the path behind you before starting. Never step backward
toward a wall, furniture, or a step.

CONFIDENCE NOTE: The ability to step backward confidently is a key recovery skill

after a forward lean. Training it deliberately means it is available when you need it.

Exercise 10: Obstacle Step-Over

Practices lifting the foot high enough to clear a low obstacle, directly training the fall-prevention skill that matters most on thresholds, door edges, and uneven ground.

Steps:

1. Place a low obstacle on the floor. Start with something about two centimeters tall.
2. Stand about one step back from the obstacle.
3. Lift your right foot higher than you think necessary and step over the obstacle.

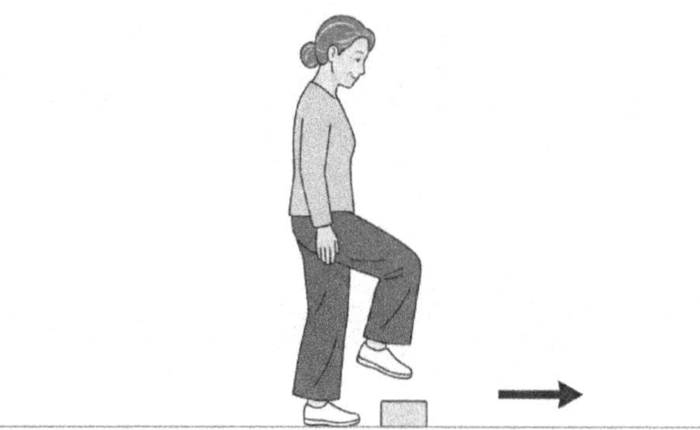

4. Place the right foot down on the other side. Pause.
5. Bring the left foot over the obstacle the same way.
6. Turn around and step back over it in the same way.
7. Complete four crossings.
8. Raise the obstacle height slightly when four crossings feel easy.

FEEL IT: A deliberate, controlled lift of each foot that clears the obstacle with room to spare. Aim for more clearance than you need.

SAFETY TIP: Do not rush. A stumble on an obstacle during practice is just as real as one on a kerb. Take each crossing slowly.

CONFIDENCE NOTE: Door thresholds, kerb edges, and garden hoses are the most common trip hazards for older adults. This exercise directly practices clearing exactly those situations.

> **MODIFICATION:**
> Begin with a flat line of tape on the floor before adding any height. The stepping-over habit is more important than the height of the obstacle.

Exercise 11: Direction-Change Walk

Practices stopping and changing walking direction cleanly, which trains the balance response needed for unpredictable real-world situations.

Steps:

1. Begin walking forward at the slow pace from Exercise 2.

2. After four steps, come to a complete stop. Stand still for two counts.

3. Turn 90 degrees to the right. Weight transferring to right foot. Left foot beginning to pivot. Take two steps in the new direction.

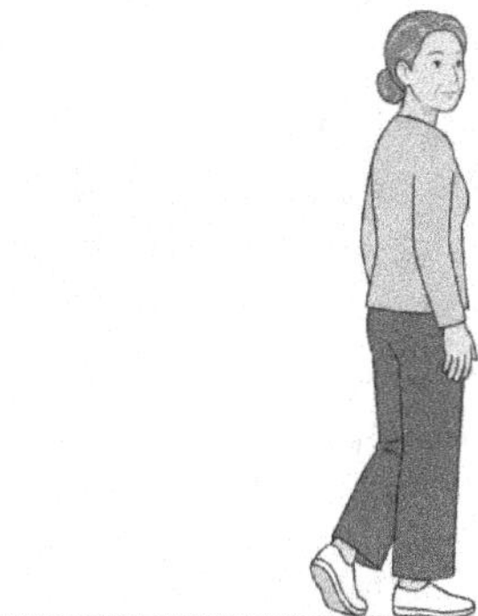

4. Stop again. Turn to face forward. Take four steps.

5. Stop again. Turn 90 degrees to the left. Weight transferring to left foot. Right foot beginning to pivot. Take two steps in the new direction.

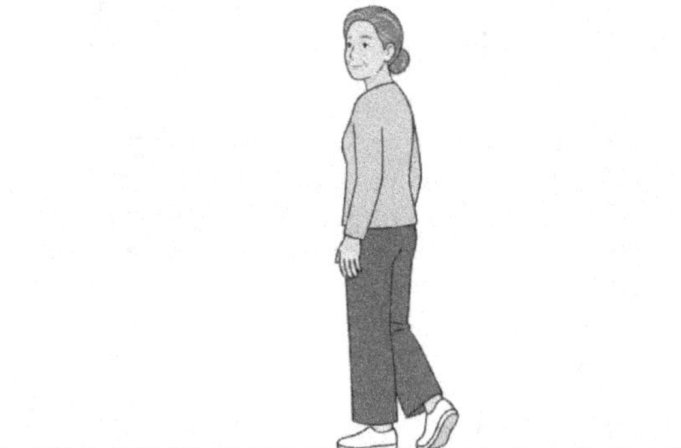

6. Stop. Turn back to your original direction. Continue.

7. Repeat the pattern twice.

FEEL IT: A clear weight transfer to the standing foot each time you stop. The stop and the turn happen separately, not simultaneously.

SAFETY TIP: Come to a full stop before turning. Turning while still walking forward is how many falls happen.

CONFIDENCE NOTE: Shops, pavements, and crowded spaces require constant stopping and direction changes. Practicing this pattern in a controlled space makes those moments much steadier.

> **MODIFICATION:**
> Reduce the turns to smaller angles (45 degrees) before working up to 90. A smaller turn is easier to manage.

Exercise 12: Confidence Walk

A full-length walking sequence that puts all the skills together without stopping to think about individual elements. This is what walking feels like when the training has taken effect.

Steps:

1. Stand at the start of your walking path.

2. Begin walking forward using everything you have practiced: heel first, deliberate pace, toes lifting, arms swinging.

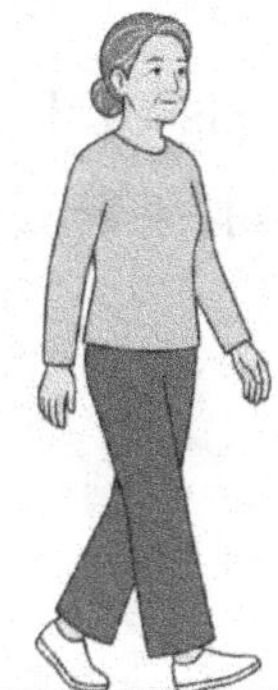

3. Walk at a pace that feels controlled but not artificially slow. This is slightly faster than Exercises 1 and 2.

4. Continue for the full length of your path.

5. At the end, turn using the direction-change method from Exercise 11.

6. Walk back at the same pace.

7. Do two full lengths.

FEEL IT: A walking pace that feels like you, but steadier. Not mechanical, not rushed. Just your natural walk, with better mechanics underneath it.

SAFETY TIP: This exercise should feel easier than Exercise 1 did when you first started. If it does not, return to the slower pace.

CONFIDENCE NOTE: This is the exercise that measures how far you have come. Use it on the first day of every week as a simple self-check.

> **MODIFICATION:**
> There is no modification needed for this exercise. If any element feels difficult, return to the individual exercise that trains it.

Common Walking Mistakes Seniors Make – and How to Fix Them

These five mistakes are the most common ones I see older adults make when they start paying attention to their walking. None of them are character flaws. All of them are habits that formed for understandable reasons. All of them can be changed.

Mistake 1: Looking Down at the Feet

WHY IT HAPPENS: When walking feels uncertain, watching the feet feels like it should help.

WHY IT MAKES THINGS WORSE: Looking down pushes the center of gravity forward, reduces the visual field for upcoming hazards, and deprives the vestibular system of the level-head position it needs to function accurately.

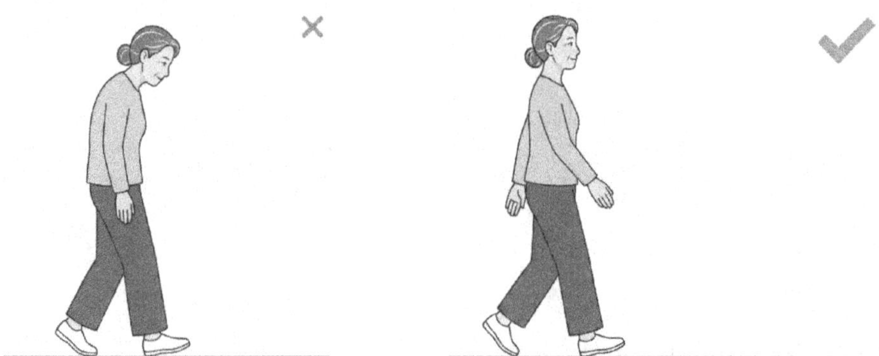

THE FIX: Before each session, find a point on the wall at eye level and use it as your gaze target. Return your eyes to this level every time you notice them dropping.

Mistake 2: Shuffling the Feet

WHY IT HAPPENS: Shuffling reduces the energy cost of lifting the feet and feels safer because the feet stay close to the ground.

WHY IT MAKES THINGS WORSE: Shuffling feet catch on the smallest irregularities: a rug edge, a slight dip, a difference between floor surfaces. Shuffling is one of the most common causes of tripping.

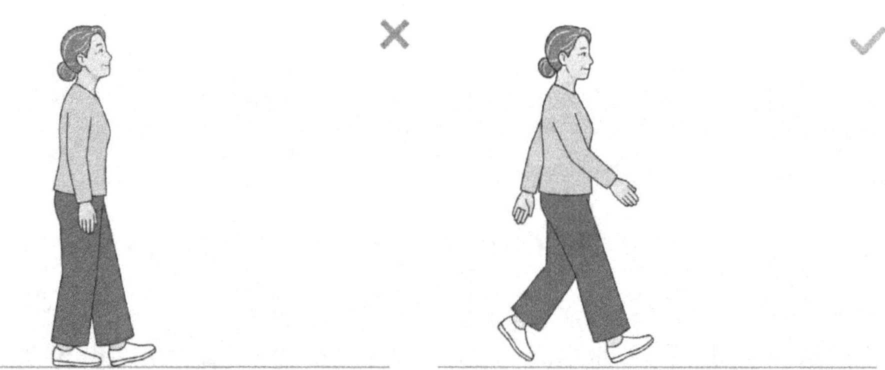

THE FIX: Practice Exercises 3 and 4 specifically. The Step and Pause and the Toe-Lift Walk directly train the habits that prevent shuffling.

Mistake 3: Holding the Arms Stiff

WHY IT HAPPENS: People who are worried about balance often brace their arms, hold them tightly at their sides, or clasp them in front.

WHY IT MAKES THINGS WORSE: Stiff arms cannot provide counterbalance. A natural arm swing acts as a stabilizer for the whole walking pattern. Removing it makes the gait less stable, not more.

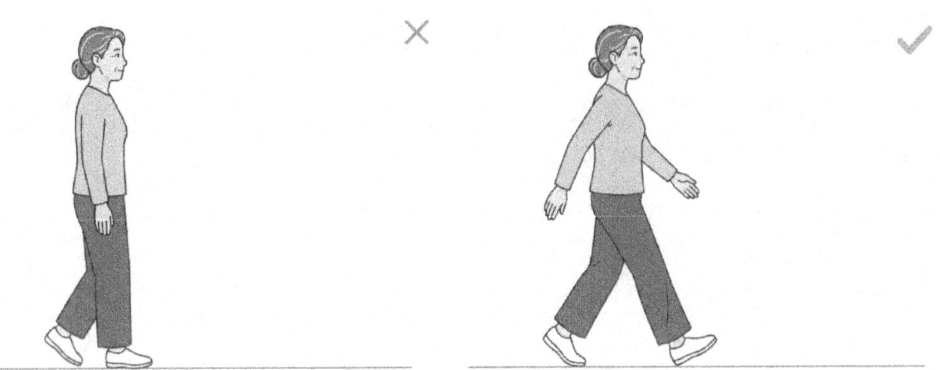

THE FIX: Practice Exercise 6 (Arm-Swing Coordination Walk) daily in Weeks Two through Four. Allow the arms to swing even if it feels unfamiliar.

Mistake 4: Taking Very Small Steps

WHY IT HAPPENS: Shorter steps feel safer because they keep the weight more evenly distributed and reduce the single-leg balance time.

WHY IT MAKES THINGS WORSE: Very short steps reduce the hip extension that keeps the gait efficient, increase the number of balance transitions per unit of distance, and actually increase fatigue.

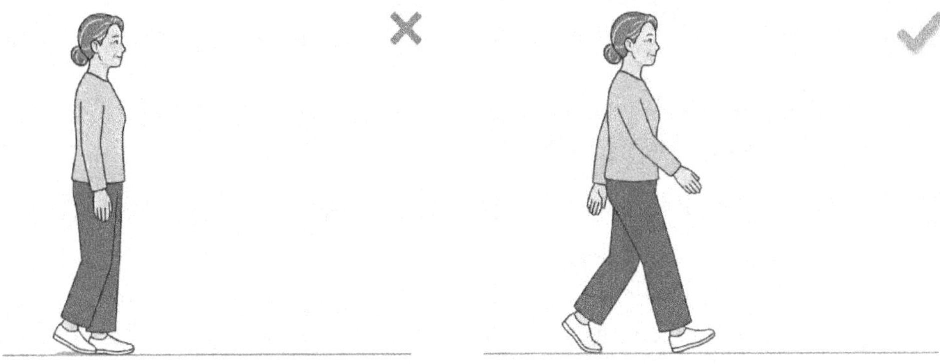

THE FIX: Use the Slow-Motion Forward Walk (Exercise 2) to practice a natural stride length at a reduced speed. As confidence grows, the stride length will return naturally.

Mistake 5: Tensing Against a Potential Fall
WHY IT HAPPENS: After a fall or a scare, the body learns to brace against the next one. Every walk is accompanied by a low level of physical tension that feels like caution but is actually preparation for impact.

WHY IT MAKES THINGS WORSE: Braced muscles cannot make the rapid, fluid micro-adjustments that balance requires. A tense walker is actually more likely to fall than a relaxed one because rigidity prevents the corrective responses.

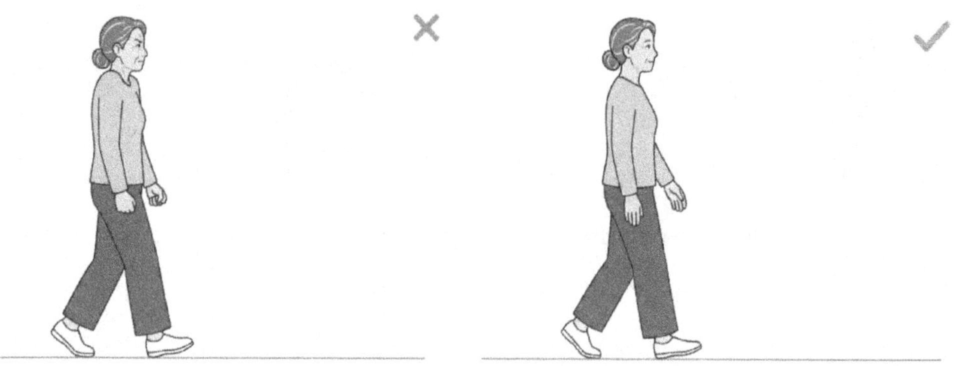

THE FIX: Before each session, take three slow breaths and consciously drop the shoulders. Do the same at the midpoint of each practice walk.

Using a Walking Aid – How to Adapt These Exercises

If you use a cane or a walking frame, all twelve exercises can be adapted. Here is how.

With a cane: keep the cane in your usual hand throughout the exercises. The exercises do not change the role of the cane, they add deliberate attention to the mechanics of the walking. For Exercise 5 (Wide-Base Side Step), move the cane out with the stepping foot to maintain your base. For Exercise 7 (Heel-to-Toe Precision Walk), use the cane for light balance support while still placing the feet in the precise position. For Exercise 9 (Backward Step and Hold), move the cane backward before the stepping foot.

With a walking frame: Exercise 2 (Slow-Motion Walk) and Exercise 1 (Grounded Heel Step) work exactly as described with the frame providing your balance support. Exercises 5, 7, and 9 are more challenging with a frame. For these, stand beside the frame and hold it with one hand while performing the exercise with a reduced range, or skip them in the early weeks and introduce them when balance has improved.

Exercise 12 (Confidence Walk) should be performed with whatever aid you normally use. The goal is confident walking, not walking without aids. A confident walk with a cane is just as valid an outcome as a confident walk without one.

A Small Request

If this book made a difference for you, even in a small way, would you consider leaving an honest review on Amazon or through the website you got a hold of this book?

As an independent author, I don't have the marketing budget of large publishing houses. Reviews are how readers discover books like this. Your feedback truly helps this work reach others who may need it.

It only takes two minutes, and your honest thoughts, positive or critical are genuinely appreciated.

You can leave your review on Amazon by searching the title ***Tai Chi Walking Exercises for Seniors Over 60 by Liuhe Chen*** on Amazon. It takes two minutes, and it matters more than you know.

Chapter 5

The 28-Day Walking Program

This is the daily program. Read each day's entry before you begin the session, including Liuhe's Note and the NOTICE TODAY prompt. They take 30 seconds to read and they change the quality of what follows.

The program is built around three goals: preventing falls, rebuilding balance, and walking with more confidence. Every session refers back to at least one of these goals. The progress checks at the end of each week help you track what is actually changing, so that Day 28 is a real record rather than a general impression. Use each check honestly, including the items that show limited progress. Those are where the remaining work is.

Session times: ten minutes in Weeks One and Two, up to twelve minutes in Weeks Three and Four. Never push past twelve minutes. The benefit comes from consistency and quality, not from extra time.

If you miss a session, do not try to make it up by doing two sessions the following day. Return to the next scheduled session and continue from there. Missing one session in a week has a minimal effect on the overall outcome. Compressing two sessions into one reduces the recovery time between training stimuli and produces less adaptation, not more.

Each week ends with a rest day and a progress check. The rest day on Day 7 comes before the check, not after, so that the check reflects a session done after a full day of consolidation. This is deliberate. The session after a rest day is almost always the best session of the week. The progress check captures the state of the practice at its best.

Week 1 – Find Your Ground

This week uses three exercises: Grounded Heel Step, Slow-Motion Forward Walk, and Step and Pause. The sessions are ten minutes. The focus is on learning to feel the ground before trusting it, to slow the pace enough that each step is under full control, and to build the single-leg balance moment that is at the heart of every safe step.

Most people find the first couple of sessions feel more mental than physical. You are learning three new movement patterns simultaneously. The effort is real. It eases by Day 4.

A common question in Week One is whether the movements should feel awkward. The answer is yes, for the first two or three sessions. Any new motor pattern feels mechanical and deliberate before it becomes fluent. If the Grounded Heel Step feels like you are thinking about every footfall, that is because you are. That deliberateness is the training. By Day 5 or 6, the heel-first landing will start to feel more natural. By the end of Week Two, it will be the new automatic.

> **What to Expect This Week**
> • Fall prevention: your heel will start to feel the floor differently within the first few sessions.
> • Balance: the Step and Pause will feel uncertain at first. That uncertainty is exactly what is being trained.
> • Confidence: keep the chair within easy reach throughout this week. It is not a crutch. It is a sensible starting point.

Day 1 – Your First Tai Chi Walk

> **SESSION AT A GLANCE**
> Duration: 10 minutes
> Exercises: Grounded Heel Step, Slow-Motion Forward Walk
> Low-energy option: Grounded Heel Step only, 5 minutes

> **Liuhe's Note:**
> Today is not about doing it perfectly. It is about learning what deliberate walking feels like compared to automatic walking. Go slowly. Notice the difference between a heel-first step and your usual step. If the session feels short, that is correct. Ten minutes of deliberate practice is more than enough for Day 1.

> **NOTICE TODAY:**
> NOTICE TODAY: As you walk, notice whether your heel touches the floor before your full weight follows. That moment is what this program is building.

> **SAFETY REMINDER:**

> Keep the chair within arm's reach throughout this session.

Day 2 – Adding the Pause

SESSION AT A GLANCE
Duration: 10 minutes
Exercises: Grounded Heel Step, Slow-Motion Forward Walk, Step and Pause
Low-energy option: Exercises 1 and 2 only

Liuhe's Note:
Exercise 3 (Step and Pause) is the hardest thing you will do in Week One. The brief balance moment during the pause is where most of the fall-prevention training lives. Be patient with it.

NOTICE TODAY:
NOTICE TODAY: During Step and Pause, notice which leg feels steadier as your standing leg. Most people have a stronger balance side. Both sides will improve.

SAFETY REMINDER:
For the Step and Pause, keep one hand close to the wall or chair in the first two sessions.

Day 3 – Rest and Recover

REST DAY
No walking session today. After two sessions of new movement patterns, your nervous system needs time to consolidate what it has learned. Rest is not wasted time. It is when the training takes hold.

Liuhe's Note:
Take a short gentle walk today if you want to move, but do not practice the exercises. Let your muscles recover with a warm bath or gentle stretching of the calves and ankles.

Day 4 – Returning to the Path

SESSION AT A GLANCE
Duration: 10 minutes
Exercises: Grounded Heel Step, Slow-Motion Walk, Step and Pause
Low-energy option: Exercises 1 and 2 only

Liuhe's Note:
Most people find the session after a rest day feels noticeably steadier. The pause in Step and Pause will probably feel a little easier today than it did on Day 2. That improvement happened during the rest, not during practice.

NOTICE TODAY:
NOTICE TODAY: As you return to the exercises, notice whether the Grounded Heel Step feels more natural than it did on Day 1.

SAFETY REMINDER:
If Day 3 rest has left you stiffer than usual, do the warm-up from Chapter Three slowly before beginning.

Day 5 – Building the Routine

SESSION AT A GLANCE
Duration: 10 minutes
Exercises: All three Week One exercises, two lengths each
Low-energy option: Exercise 1 and one length of Exercise 3

Liuhe's Note:
By Day 5 the three exercises should feel familiar enough that you are not thinking about each step as a sequence. You can start thinking about the quality of each step: how solidly the heel lands, how steady the pause is.

NOTICE TODAY:
NOTICE TODAY: Walk the full session and ask yourself at the end: did any step feel genuinely confident? Name one.

SAFETY REMINDER:
The Step and Pause can become slightly faster as familiarity increases. Resist the urge to rush it.

Day 6 – Rest and Recover

REST DAY
Second rest day this week. Two sessions of deliberate walking practice and one rest day is the pattern that produces the best balance improvement. Today the balance system is making the neural adaptations that tomorrow's practice will build on.

Liuhe's Note:
Drink extra water today. Joint fluid, which this program is helping to circulate, is water-based.
Gentle ankle circles while sitting are a useful way to keep the joint lubricated on rest days.

Day 7 – Week One Progress Check

SESSION AT A GLANCE
Duration: 10 minutes
Exercises: Grounded Heel Step, Slow-Motion Walk, Step and Pause
Focus: awareness of change since Day 1

Liuhe's Note:
Walk the full session as you normally would, then complete the progress check below while
the session is still fresh. Compare honestly to Day 1, not to an ideal.

NOTICE TODAY:
NOTICE TODAY: Complete the full session, then sit and complete the progress check while
the walk is still fresh in your body.

SAFETY REMINDER:
No new safety requirements today. Continue as in previous sessions.

PROGRESS CHECK
End of Week One. Compare your experience today to Day 1. Use the checkboxes below.

FALL PREVENTION: Does the heel land before the weight follows more of the time than on
Day 1? a) Yes b) Sometimes c) Not yet
BALANCE: Is the pause in Step and Pause steadier than it was on Day 2? a) Yes, noticeably
b) Slightly c) About the same
CONFIDENCE: Did you keep the chair within reach throughout this week? a) Yes, I still
need it b) I moved a step further away c) I rarely needed it
OVERALL: Did you complete all five practice sessions? a) All five b) Four c) Three or
fewer

YOUR OBSERVATION: Write one specific change you noticed this week:

Week Two adds three new exercises and brings in arm coordination and sideways stepping.
You will start to feel the balance work in new areas, particularly the outer hips.

Week 2 – Build Your Balance

Week Two uses six exercises: the three from Week One, plus Toe-Lift Walk, Wide-Base Side Step, and Arm-Swing Coordination Walk. Sessions remain ten minutes. Three new exercises come in, but you keep the old ones. The program never drops what you have learned, it builds on it.

The focus this week is on balance from all directions, not just forward. The side step challenges the outer hip stabilizers. The arm swing restores the whole-body coordination that cautious walking has reduced. The toe lift directly reduces the trip risk.

One thing to watch in Week Two is the tendency to rush through the earlier exercises to get to the new ones. Exercises 1 through 3 from Week One are still doing important work. The heel landing and the pause are the foundation that all six exercises this week are built on. Give them the same attention you did in Week One, not less.

By the middle of Week Two, the routine of a daily practice session should be starting to settle. The setup, the warm-up, the exercises, the close: this sequence will feel more familiar by Day 11 or 12 than it did on Day 8. That familiarity is the habit forming. It is one of the most valuable outcomes of the first two weeks.

What to Expect This Week
- Fall prevention: the toe-lift exercise will make your foot clearance more reliable. You may notice it carry over into your ordinary daily walking within a few sessions.
- Balance: the wide-base side step will feel harder than it looks. The outer hip doing its job is not a comfortable sensation at first.
- Confidence: six exercises is a lot to hold in mind. Do not rush through them. A slower, careful session with all six is better than a fast incomplete one.

Day 8 – Three New Exercises

SESSION AT A GLANCE
Duration: 10 minutes
Exercises: All six Week Two exercises, one length or set each
Low-energy option: Exercises 1, 2, 3 from Week One only

Liuhe's Note:

Three new exercises today. Read through Exercises 4, 5, and 6 in Chapter Four before this session if you have not already. Practice each new one separately before trying to link them all.

NOTICE TODAY:
NOTICE TODAY: During the Wide-Base Side Step, notice which direction feels less steady. That is the side to focus on.

SAFETY REMINDER:
The side step is a new direction of movement. Keep a wall or chair within easy reach for the first time you practice it.

Day 9 – Linking the Six

SESSION AT A GLANCE
Duration: 10 minutes
Exercises: All six, two lengths/sets each
Low-energy option: Any four exercises that feel most useful today

Liuhe's Note:
Now that the new exercises are slightly familiar, focus on linking them smoothly one after another. You should be spending about ninety seconds on each exercise.

NOTICE TODAY:
NOTICE TODAY: Notice whether the arm swing in Exercise 6 makes the walk feel more or less stable than Exercise 2 without arm swing.

SAFETY REMINDER:
Toe-lift walking tires the shin muscles faster than normal. Stop the exercise before you feel the foot dragging.

Day 10 – Rest and Recover

REST DAY
Rest day. Your outer hip muscles are likely feeling the side step work from the past two sessions. This is normal soreness from muscles being used in a new way. Rest lets them adapt.

Liuhe's Note:

If the outer hips feel sore, gentle seated hip circles (sitting in a chair and rotating each knee slowly outward and back) can help maintain circulation without adding training load.

Day 11 – Balance Focus

SESSION AT A GLANCE
Duration: 10 minutes
Exercises: All six, with extra time on Exercises 3 and 5
Low-energy option: Exercises 1, 3, 5 only

Liuhe's Note:
Today give the Step and Pause and the Wide-Base Side Step a little extra attention. These are the two exercises doing the most direct balance work in Week Two. Quality in these two carries the most benefit. For the side step, focus on keeping the hips level as the weight shifts. A dropping hip on the stepping side is the most common form error.

NOTICE TODAY:
NOTICE TODAY: In the Step and Pause, count the seconds of the pause on your weaker balance side. Even a small increase from Day 2 is real progress.

SAFETY REMINDER:
During the side step, make sure the feet point forward throughout. Toes turning out is the most common form error and reduces the hip training effect.

Day 12 – Coordination Day

SESSION AT A GLANCE
Duration: 10 minutes
Exercises: All six, emphasis on Exercise 6
Low-energy option: Exercises 1, 2, 6

Liuhe's Note:
The Arm-Swing Coordination Walk (Exercise 6) often feels awkward for the first few sessions and then suddenly clicks into a rhythm. Today, if you feel the click, stay with it for an extra length.

NOTICE TODAY:
NOTICE TODAY: Does the arm-swing walk feel more natural today than it did on Day 8? Any improvement in coordination fluency is your nervous system consolidating the pattern.

SAFETY REMINDER:
Walking with arm swing uses more space than walking with arms at sides. Make sure your path is clear before starting.

Day 13 – Rest and Recover

REST DAY
Second rest day of Week Two. Five sessions of balance training this week. Your nervous system has been working hard. Tonight's sleep is when the largest part of the balance improvement will be consolidated.

Liuhe's Note:
Prioritize good sleep tonight. The neural pathways being built by this program are strengthened during slow-wave sleep. A full night's sleep after a practice week is worth more than an extra session.

Day 14 – Week Two Progress Check

SESSION AT A GLANCE
Duration: 10 minutes
Exercises: All six Week Two exercises
Focus: measurement of progress

Liuhe's Note:
Walk all six exercises today with full attention. After the session, compare your experience to your Week One check. The outer hip soreness from side stepping should be less this week.

NOTICE TODAY:
NOTICE TODAY: Walk Exercise 12 (Confidence Walk) even though it is not formally in your week yet. Use it as an informal test of how your walking feels compared to Day 1.

SAFETY REMINDER:
No new safety requirements this week. Continue as normal.

PROGRESS CHECK
End of Week Two. Compare to your Week One check and your Day 1 starting point.

FALL PREVENTION: Is the toe lift in Exercise 4 becoming more automatic, or does it still need conscious effort? a) More automatic b) Still conscious c) Inconsistent

BALANCE: Has the pause in Step and Pause become steadier on your weaker side? a) Yes b) Slightly c) About the same

CONFIDENCE: Are you walking further from the chair or wall than in Week One? a) Yes, notably further b) A little further c) About the same

SIDE STEP: Is the outer hip discomfort from Wide-Base Side Step less than it was on Day 8? a) Yes, much less b) Slightly less c) About the same

YOUR OBSERVATION: Write one specific improvement you have noticed in your ordinary daily walking:

Week Three adds three more exercises including the figure-eight path and backward stepping. Sessions increase to ten to twelve minutes. You will start working on direction changes and obstacle awareness.

Week 3 – Walk with Control

Week Three uses nine exercises: all six from Week Two, plus Heel-to-Toe Precision Walk, Figure-Eight Walking Path, and Backward Step and Hold. Sessions run ten to twelve minutes. This week asks more of your attention because the new exercises require spatial awareness that the earlier ones did not.

The confidence theme begins in earnest this week. The figure-eight path practices real-world turning. The backward step builds the recovery skill you need for forward stumbles. The heel-to-toe walk challenges balance in a narrower, more demanding pattern than any exercise so far.

Some people find Week Three the most rewarding and the most frustrating week of the program in equal measure. The new exercises are genuinely hard. The heel-to-toe walk in particular is uncomfortable for people who have been walking cautiously for some time. That discomfort is information: it tells you exactly where the balance system is being stretched. Stay with the discomfort if it is the productive kind. Use the wall for support but keep practicing.

The confidence changes this week tend to appear outside the sessions rather than within them. After two weeks of heel-landing practice, people start to notice the heel contacting the floor on ordinary walks without having to think about it. After two weeks of side stepping, a sideways stumble catch feels slightly more available. These small carry-overs are the program working at the neural level, exactly as intended.

> **What to Expect This Week**
> • Fall prevention: the obstacle step-over (introduced in Week Four) is built on the foot-lift habits you are reinforcing this week. Every clean toe lift now makes that exercise easier later.
> • Balance: the heel-to-toe walk will feel genuinely difficult at first. That is the point. Narrow-line balance is the hardest balance demand in daily life.
> • Confidence: completing all nine exercises in one session is an achievement. Give yourself credit for it.

Day 15 – Three More Exercises

> **SESSION AT A GLANCE**
> Duration: 10-12 minutes
> Exercises: All nine Week Three exercises, one set/length each
> Low-energy option: Six Week Two exercises only

> **Liuhe's Note:**
> Read through Exercises 7, 8, and 9 in Chapter Four before this session. Exercise 8 (Figure-Eight) requires setting up two floor markers. Have them ready before you start.

> **NOTICE TODAY:**
> NOTICE TODAY: During the Figure-Eight walk, notice whether turning to the right or to the left feels more natural. Most people have a preferred direction.

> **SAFETY REMINDER:**
> The Backward Step (Exercise 9) requires clear space behind you. Check the path before starting.

Day 16 – Precision and Control

> **SESSION AT A GLANCE**
> Duration: 10-12 minutes
> Exercises: All nine, emphasis on Exercises 7 and 8
> Low-energy option: Any six exercises

> **Liuhe's Note:**
> The Heel-to-Toe Precision Walk is the single most balance-demanding exercise in the program. If it feels very hard today, that is expected. Use wall support and reduce the number of steps rather than skipping it.

NOTICE TODAY:
NOTICE TODAY: In the heel-to-toe walk, count how many steps you take before you need to touch the wall. Write down the number. It will increase.

SAFETY REMINDER:
Always have a wall or chair within touching distance during the heel-to-toe walk.

Day 17 – Rest and Recover

REST DAY
Rest day. Week Three is the most challenging week in the program. Two days of nine exercises is significant training volume. Today the balance adaptations are consolidating.

Liuhe's Note:
This is a good day to re-read the safety and modification notes for any exercise that felt difficult this week. Knowing the modification means you can use it confidently rather than just stopping.

Day 18 – Turning and Recovery

SESSION AT A GLANCE
Duration: 10-12 minutes
Exercises: All nine, with extra attention on Exercises 8 and 9
Low-energy option: Exercises 1-6 plus Exercise 8

Liuhe's Note:
The Figure-Eight and Backward Step are this week's confidence builders. Both directly train the movements that matter most in unpredictable situations. Give them real attention today.

NOTICE TODAY:
NOTICE TODAY: During the Backward Step, notice how the weight shifts differ from forward walking. The backward landing is on the ball of the foot first.

SAFETY REMINDER:
For the backward step, count your steps aloud to maintain awareness of how far back you are going.

Day 19 – Full Control Session

SESSION AT A GLANCE
Duration: 10-12 minutes
Exercises: All nine in sequence
Low-energy option: Any five exercises of your choice

Liuhe's Note:
Today try running all nine exercises in sequence without stopping between them. The transition from one exercise to the next is part of the training. Notice how the balance demand changes with each exercise. You should find that some transitions feel easy and some require a moment of mental shifting. The difficult transitions are where the most neural work is happening.

NOTICE TODAY:
NOTICE TODAY: How does walking feel at the end of a nine-exercise session compared to how it felt at the start of Day 1?

SAFETY REMINDER:
At twelve minutes, stop regardless of where you are in the sequence. The time limit is there for a reason.

Day 20 – Rest and Recover

REST DAY
Second rest day of Week Three. Five sessions of increasingly demanding balance work this week. Rest is especially important this week because the new exercises have been asking more of your balance system than any previous week.

Liuhe's Note:
Notice how your ordinary walking feels today, on the rest day. Many people find that rest days are when they first notice the practice carrying over into daily movement.

Day 21 – Week Three Progress Check

SESSION AT A GLANCE
Duration: 10-12 minutes
Exercises: All nine Week Three exercises
Focus: comparison and measurement

Liuhe's Note:
Walk the full nine-exercise session. After the session, complete the progress check while the session is still fresh.

NOTICE TODAY:
NOTICE TODAY: After the session, walk to a different room in your home. Notice whether anything about how that ordinary walk feels has changed since Day 1.

SAFETY REMINDER:
No new requirements. Continue as normal.

PROGRESS CHECK
End of Week Three. Compare to Week Two and to Day 1.

CONFIDENCE: Did you attempt the heel-to-toe walk without wall support for any part of the session? a) Yes, for several steps b) I used the wall lightly c) I still need full support
BALANCE: Is the figure-eight walking path feeling smoother than it did on Day 15? a) Yes, noticeably b) A little c) About the same
FALL PREVENTION: Has the backward step become more confident than it was on Day 15? a) Yes b) Somewhat c) Still building
DAILY LIFE: Have you noticed any improvement in how you walk during ordinary daily activities? a) Yes, specifically: b) Not yet

YOUR OBSERVATION: Name the single exercise that has improved most since you first tried it:

Week Four completes the program with all twelve exercises. You will add obstacle stepping and the Confidence Walk, and each session will bring everything together into a continuous practice.

Week 4 – Walk with Confidence

Week Four uses all twelve exercises. Sessions run ten to twelve minutes. The three new exercises are Obstacle Step-Over, Direction-Change Walk, and Confidence Walk. This week the program asks you to put everything together and to start applying it to real-world walking situations.

The confidence theme is not a reassurance. It is a practical target. By Day 28, you should have specific evidence of improved walking confidence: a situation you handle better, a place you walk to more readily, a step you take without the hesitation that would have been there in Week One.

The twelve exercises together take ten to twelve minutes, which means roughly one minute per exercise on average. The sequence flows: walking exercises flow into balance exercises into confidence exercises. If you find yourself stopping and starting between exercises, try to reduce the pause to just a breath or two. A smooth session is more effective than a choppy one.

What to Expect This Week
• Fall prevention: the obstacle step-over is the exercise most directly related to the kind of trips that happen in real life. Practice it with real attention.
• Balance: twelve exercises is the full program. Getting through all twelve in twelve minutes requires a smooth, unhurried pace throughout.
• Confidence: use the Confidence Walk on Day 22 as a measure of where you are now, and again on Day 28 as your final assessment.

Day 22 – All Twelve

SESSION AT A GLANCE
Duration: 10-12 minutes
Exercises: All twelve, one set/length each
Low-energy option: Any nine exercises of your choice

Liuhe's Note:
Two new exercises today: Obstacle Step-Over and Direction-Change Walk. Read both in Chapter Four before starting. Set up a small floor obstacle before the session begins. For the Direction-Change Walk, plan your turning points before the session starts so you are not improvising the route mid-walk. Knowing where the turns are lets you focus on how you make them.

NOTICE TODAY:
NOTICE TODAY: After today's Confidence Walk (Exercise 12), notice how it compares to how walking felt on Day 1. Something specific will have changed.

SAFETY REMINDER:
For the Obstacle Step-Over, start with the lowest possible obstacle height. There is no benefit to using a high obstacle.

Day 23 – Integration

> **SESSION AT A GLANCE**
> Duration: 10-12 minutes
> Exercises: All twelve in sequence
> Low-energy option: Any eight exercises

> **Liuhe's Note:**
> Today focus on transitions between exercises rather than on individual exercise quality. Moving smoothly from one to the next is itself a balance skill.

> **NOTICE TODAY:**
> NOTICE TODAY: Notice whether the Direction-Change Walk feels easier or harder than the Figure-Eight walk from Exercise 8. Both train turning, but in different ways.

> **SAFETY REMINDER:**
> Check floor space before every session. Twelve exercises need more space than three.

Day 24 – Rest and Recover

> **REST DAY**
> Rest day. Two days of the full twelve-exercise program is the most demanding training load of the program. The rest today is essential for consolidating the Week Four adaptations.

> **Liuhe's Note:**
> Take a short gentle walk outdoors if the weather allows. After three weeks of deliberate training, ordinary outdoor walking will probably feel different. Notice how.

Day 25 – Real-World Application

> **SESSION AT A GLANCE**
> Duration: 10-12 minutes
> Exercises: All twelve
> Focus: thinking about real-world walking situations

> **Liuhe's Note:**
> Today as you practice each exercise, think about where it applies in your real walking life. The obstacle step-over: think of a threshold you cross daily. The direction-change walk: think of a

corner you turn regularly. The Confidence Walk: think of a specific place you want to walk more easily. The exercises are the training. The real walk is the point.

NOTICE TODAY:
NOTICE TODAY: Is there a specific real-world walking situation that feels more manageable this week than it did four weeks ago? Name it.

SAFETY REMINDER:
Maintain the slow deliberate pace even in the final week. Speed is not the goal.

Day 26 – Confidence Session

SESSION AT A GLANCE
Duration: 10-12 minutes
Exercises: All twelve, emphasis on Exercises 10, 11, 12
Low-energy option: Exercises 10, 11, 12 plus any three from earlier weeks

Liuhe's Note:
The last three exercises are the confidence exercises. Today give them the most time. Exercise 12 (Confidence Walk) at the end should feel like a demonstration of everything you have built, not just another drill. If the Confidence Walk still feels mechanical rather than natural, that is fine. Some people need more than 28 days for the full integration. What matters is that it is better than Day 1.

NOTICE TODAY:
NOTICE TODAY: Walk Exercise 12 last. As you walk, notice whether you are thinking about each step or whether the walking is flowing more automatically.

SAFETY REMINDER:
Two days left. Trust what you have built. The training is in the body now.

Day 27 – Rest and Recover

REST DAY
Final rest day of the program. Tomorrow is Day 28. Today the body and brain are making the last round of adaptations before the final assessment.

Liuhe's Note:

Spend a few minutes today thinking about three things: one walk that felt different this week compared to Week One, one situation you handle with more confidence, and one exercise that surprised you with how much it improved.

Day 28 – Your Final Walk

SESSION AT A GLANCE
Duration: 10-12 minutes
Exercises: All twelve in full
Focus: complete final walk and Day 28 progress review

Liuhe's Note:
Walk the full program today. End with Exercise 12 and let it be a proper walk at a pace that feels like your walk, not a drill. After the session, complete the final progress check before doing anything else. Write the answers in full sentences where the checkboxes invite them. The words you use will tell you something about what actually changed.

NOTICE TODAY:
NOTICE TODAY: As you walk Exercise 12 for the last session, ask yourself: is this the same walk you did on Day 1? In what specific way is it different?

SAFETY REMINDER:
Complete the session fully before reading the progress check. The walk is the evidence. The check is just the record.

PROGRESS CHECK
Day 28. The full program is complete. Compare honestly to Day 1 and to your previous weekly checks.

FALL PREVENTION: Does the heel land before the weight follows more of the time in ordinary daily walking (not just in sessions)? a) Yes, reliably b) Sometimes c) Still mostly in sessions only
BALANCE: Has the Step and Pause improved on both sides since Day 2? a) Yes, both sides b) One side more than the other c) About the same
CONFIDENCE: Is there a specific real-world walking situation that you handle more confidently than on Day 1? a) Yes, specifically: b) Not yet specific c) Not yet
OBSTACLE STEP: Can you step over a low obstacle without slowing to almost a stop? a) Yes b) I slow down less than before c) Still working on it
OVERALL: What is the single most important change your walking has made in 28 days? Write:

Read Chapter Eight for guidance on how to read these results honestly and how to build on them. The 28 days are the foundation. What you do after Day 28 determines how far the improvement goes.

Chapter 6

Eating, Resting, and Looking After Your Joints

The ten minutes of walking practice each day does the training. What you eat, how you sleep, and how you manage your joints in the other twenty-three hours and fifty minutes determines how well that training takes. This chapter covers the key factors in plain terms, without requiring any dramatic changes to your existing habits.

What Your Joints Need to Keep Moving Well

The joints of the ankles, knees, and hips do the most work in walking. They are cushioned by cartilage and lubricated by synovial fluid, and both of these require specific conditions to stay in good working order.

The joints that bear the most load in walking are the ankles, knees, and hips. Each of these is enclosed in a joint capsule that produces synovial fluid and houses cartilage surfaces that rely entirely on movement for their nutrition. Understanding how these joints work makes the exercises in this program easier to do with the right quality of attention.

Cartilage has no blood supply. The only way nutrients reach it and waste products leave it is through the compression and release of movement. When you walk slowly and deliberately, you are delivering exactly this loading and unloading to the joint cartilage. A joint that is regularly moved through its range stays better nourished than one that is rarely used. This is one of the reasons regular gentle walking is better for arthritic joints than rest, despite what the discomfort might suggest.

Synovial fluid, the joint's natural lubricant, is produced by the lining of the joint and works in the same way as cartilage nutrition: it distributes through the joint when the joint moves. A joint that has been still overnight, such as first thing in the morning, has less well-distributed synovial fluid than one that has been moving. This is why morning stiffness is so common. The warm-up routine in Chapter Three, done before each session, kickstarts the synovial circulation in the main walking joints so they are ready for the practice.

Two things reduce joint fluid quality: dehydration and inflammation. Both are within your control. Dehydration is the most commonly overlooked contributor to joint stiffness. Synovial fluid is partly water-based. When the body is mildly dehydrated, as many older adults chronically are, the fluid becomes thicker and less effective. Drinking enough water is a direct joint health measure. The target is roughly six to eight glasses a day for most people, more in warm weather or after exercise.

A simple way to assess your hydration is urine color: pale yellow indicates good hydration, dark yellow or amber indicates mild dehydration. Making it a habit to drink a glass of water before and after each walking session is an easy way to ensure the joints are as well-lubricated as possible for the practice and for the recovery afterward.

Cold weather reduces the awareness of thirst more than warm weather does. Older adults in cool climates or air-conditioned environments may be chronically mildly dehydrated without realizing it because they do not feel thirsty. If you notice that your joints feel stiffer than usual in the morning, increasing fluid intake is one of the simplest things to try before any other intervention.

Foods That Support Balance and Bone Strength

You do not need a special diet to support this walking program. But some straightforward food choices consistently help the body manage what the walking is training.

Protein is the building material for muscle. Every exercise in this program is asking your leg muscles to do more precise work than they normally do. Without adequate protein, those muscles cannot repair and strengthen between sessions. For most older adults, the target is around half a gram of protein per pound of body weight per day. In practical terms, this means a serving of fish, chicken, eggs, dairy, beans, or tofu at most meals. Spreading protein across the day matters more than the total amount, because the body can only use a limited amount of protein for muscle building in any single meal.

Calcium and vitamin D are the two nutrients most directly related to bone strength. Strong bones support the walking exercises, and the ankle, knee, and hip joints that bear body weight all require a solid bony foundation to function well. Dairy products, leafy green vegetables, and fortified foods provide calcium. Vitamin D comes mainly from sunlight and from oily fish. Many older adults are low in vitamin D, particularly those who spend most of their time indoors. If you have not had your vitamin D levels checked recently, it is worth asking your doctor about it.

Omega-3 fatty acids, found in oily fish like salmon, mackerel, and sardines, reduce joint inflammation. Chronically inflamed joints are stiffer and more painful than healthy ones. Reducing the background inflammation through diet directly supports the joint mobility that this program is building. Two servings of oily fish per week is a reasonable and achievable target.

Anti-inflammatory foods more broadly, berries, leafy greens, olive oil, and whole grains, contribute to the same goal. You do not need to overhaul your diet. Adding two or three of these consistently makes a real difference over four weeks. Reducing processed foods, sugar, and alcohol, which all promote inflammation, is the other half of the same strategy.

Magnesium is a mineral worth a specific mention because it plays a direct role in muscle function and is commonly deficient in older adults. Muscle cramps during or after walking sessions are often a sign of magnesium deficiency. Nuts, seeds, leafy greens, and whole grains are the best food sources. If cramping is a persistent issue, speak with your doctor about whether supplementation is appropriate.

How Rest and Sleep Support Your Walking

The walking exercises in this program train the nervous system. Neural adaptation, the process by which the balance pathways in the brain become faster and more reliable, happens primarily during sleep. The practice session opens the door. Sleep is when the adaptation walks through it.

Slow-wave sleep, the deepest part of the sleep cycle, is when motor memory consolidation occurs. The heel-to-toe pattern, the pause in Step and Pause, the arm-leg coordination of Exercise 6: all of these motor programs are strengthened during slow-wave sleep. This is why the session before a rest day is often not the best session of the week, but the session after a rest day almost always is. The rest day allows a full night of consolidation that the previous session triggered. The improvement is not imagined. It is the direct product of the rest.

Getting consistent sleep matters more than the total hours for this kind of training. Going to bed and waking at roughly the same time each day, including the rest days, maintains the sleep architecture that consolidation depends on. Irregular sleep disrupts slow-wave sleep disproportionately, and the balance training loses some of its overnight consolidation benefit.

If sleep has been difficult, the walking program itself is one of the most reliable non-pharmacological aids available. Moderate daily exercise is one of the best-studied interventions for sleep quality in older adults. After two to three weeks of daily practice, most people report that sleep is noticeably easier and that morning stiffness resolves faster. The walking is training the balance system and improving the sleep that consolidates it, simultaneously.

Alcohol disrupts sleep architecture even in small amounts, particularly the deep slow-wave sleep that motor consolidation depends on. If you have been relying on a glass of wine or a small drink to get to sleep, consider reducing or eliminating it during this program. The sleep you get without alcohol tends to be deeper and more restorative, and the balance improvements from the walking will consolidate more reliably. This is not a permanent requirement. It is a four-week experiment worth trying.

The rest days in this program are scheduled deliberately. Day 3 and Day 6 in Week One bracket the two most cognitively demanding sessions, when new motor programs are being built from scratch. Day 10 and Day 13 in Week Two allow the outer hip muscles to recover from the side-step work while the balance consolidation continues. Day 17 and Day 20 in Week Three give the more demanding balance exercises time to settle. Day 24 and Day 27 in Week Four ensure the final phase of the program is building on fully recovered neural and muscular resources. Skipping any of these rest days does not add to the training. It reduces the quality of the adaptations the training produces.

Managing Pain and Stiffness Between Sessions

Some degree of muscle soreness after the first few sessions of any new exercise program is normal. The specific muscles most likely to feel it in this program are the calf muscles (from toe-lift walking), the outer hips (from side stepping), and the shin muscles (also from toe lifting). This soreness is productive: it indicates that the muscles are adapting to new demands.

The difference between productive soreness and a warning pain is usually one of location and character. Productive soreness is in the muscle belly, feels like tiredness or aching, and eases with gentle movement. Warning pain is sharp, located at or in a joint rather than in the muscle, and gets worse with movement rather than better. If you are unsure which category something falls into, rest that day and reassess. If the pain is still present the following morning, contact your doctor before continuing.

Heat and gentle movement are the most reliable tools for managing stiffness between sessions. A warm shower or a heat pack on the stiff area before the morning session helps the synovial fluid circulate and the muscles warm up. Gentle ankle circles, knee bends, and hip rotations done while seated or lying in bed in the morning take two minutes and reduce the time it takes for morning stiffness to ease.

Over-the-counter anti-inflammatory medications can help with joint pain if your doctor approves their use for you. If you are managing chronic joint pain with medication, continue to follow your doctor's guidance and use this program as a complement to, not a replacement for, their treatment plan. The exercises here are gentle enough to be compatible with most joint conditions, but your doctor knows your specific situation and should be part of any decision about pain management.

Footwear deserves a specific mention in the context of joint care. Walking shoes with thick cushioning feel comfortable but significantly reduce the sensory information reaching your feet from the ground, which is the information that proprioception depends on. A flat or minimally cushioned shoe with a firm sole allows the foot to feel the surface more accurately. If you have been wearing very thick-soled shoes, consider transitioning to a thinner sole gradually over the course of the program. Your feet will be more sensitive and more effective at reading the ground, which directly supports fall prevention.

One final note on pacing: the ten-minute session limit in this program is not a suggestion. It is a prescription. More walking practice is not better in the early weeks. The nervous system needs the rest periods between sessions to consolidate what it has learned. Pushing past ten to twelve minutes reduces the quality of the next day's session more than it adds to today's. Stay within the time limits, particularly in Weeks One and Two. By Week Four, your body will have adapted enough that you can assess how it feels and extend gently if appropriate, but the program as written does not require it.

Another pacing note: if a session feels particularly difficult on a given day, due to poor sleep, minor illness, or general fatigue, use the low-energy option listed in the Session At a Glance box. Doing a shorter, easier session on a difficult day is better than skipping entirely. Consistency across the 28 days matters more than any individual session being performed at full capacity. The program is designed to be done every practice day, including the difficult ones. A five-minute session on a hard day is not failure. It is exactly the kind of resilient consistency that builds lasting habits.

Chapter 7

Walking Safely in the Real World

The exercises in this program are the training ground. The real world is where the training gets used. This chapter covers the situations that older adults most commonly find challenging and explains how the skills you have built apply to each of them.

Stairs, Slopes, and Uneven Ground

Stairs are where many older adults feel the most acute drop in confidence. They concentrate the single-leg balance demand, the foot clearance demand, and the visual monitoring challenge into a very small space and a very specific sequence. After four weeks of this program, you have been training every one of these elements. The Grounded Heel Step, the Step and Pause, the Toe-Lift Walk, and the Obstacle Step-Over all build the specific skills that stairs require.

Going up stairs: approach the first step at your deliberate Tai Chi pace, not your normal walking speed. Place the heel of the leading foot on the step first. Press through the heel as the weight transfers. Keep the standing knee slightly bent rather than locking it as you rise. Use the handrail as a balance reference, not as a support that carries your weight. Your legs are doing the work. The rail is there to confirm, not to carry.

Going down stairs is where most stair-related falls happen, because the eccentric muscle demand, the muscles working while lengthening rather than shortening, is higher going down than up. The foot placement requires more precision. Slow down more than feels necessary. Lower the leading foot to the next step with the toes pointing slightly down, not flat. Let the ball of the foot contact first, then the heel. Maintain contact with the handrail throughout. If you are carrying anything, put it down first rather than negotiating a staircase with occupied hands.

Slopes are easier than stairs but require a specific adjustment in walking mechanics. Going uphill, the natural tendency is to lean into the slope from the waist, which rounds the upper back and reduces the effectiveness of each push-off step. Instead, keep the spine upright and let the whole body angle slightly forward from the ankles, not from the waist. The push-off from the back foot is doing more work on a slope. The calf muscles that the Toe-Lift Walk has been strengthening are the primary muscles for this push.

Going downhill, slow down before the slope begins, not after you are already on it. Shorten the step length significantly. Lean very slightly back from the hips, not from the waist or upper back. This keeps the weight over the rear foot during the transfer and reduces the forward momentum that leads to stumbles on descents. Keep the knees slightly bent and active throughout. A locked knee on a downhill slope is a direct fall risk.

Uneven ground requires the proprioceptive training you have been building throughout the program. The key is to reduce your pace even further than the Tai Chi practice pace when the ground becomes unpredictable, and to look ahead at the surface several steps in front rather than watching your feet. The feet read the ground through the sole. The eyes need to be preparing for what is coming, not monitoring what is already happening. After four weeks of deliberate heel-to-ground practice, your feet are better equipped to read the surface than they were on Day 1.

Grass is worth a specific note. Walking on grass looks simple but is proprioceptively demanding because the surface gives slightly and unevenly with each step. The heel does not contact a firm surface and the ankle has to manage small lateral variations that pavement does not present. Introduce grass walking in Week Three or Four of the program at the deliberate practice pace, not at your ordinary walking speed. A familiar lawn is the right starting point before unfamiliar outdoor ground.

Walking in Busy Places

Busy environments combine several of the most demanding walking challenges at once: unpredictable direction changes from other people, floor surface changes between areas of a shop, the cognitive load of navigating and shopping simultaneously, and the social pressure to move at a pace that may be faster than is safe.

The most important skill in a busy space is permission to walk at your own pace. Other people in a shop are not in a hurry. They move in all directions and at varying speeds. The person walking at a deliberate, controlled pace is not the problem. The person who rushes to keep up with a pace that does not match their balance is.

In a supermarket or shop, use the trolley or basket as a deliberate balance support rather than just a carrying tool. Both hands on the trolley handle provides a significant balance base. This is not a sign of weakness. It is sensible use of an available support that makes the shopping trip safer and more comfortable. Walk the trolley slowly. The aisles narrow in some sections and the floor surface changes near refrigeration units. Notice these changes and slow down at them.

Car parks are consistently rated as one of the most anxiety-inducing walking environments for older adults with balance concerns. The reasons are clear: the surface is often slightly sloped, the lighting can be poor, the markings can be confusing, and there is moving traffic. The most practical approach is to park as close to the entrance as possible, accept that this takes more time, and walk in the areas furthest from moving vehicles whenever possible. Give yourself more time than you think you need. The anxiety of being rushed in a car park produces exactly the physical tension that makes walking less safe.

Walking With Confidence After a Fall or a Scare

A fall, or even a serious stumble that was caught, changes something in the nervous system. The experience is stored as a threat memory, and the body responds to any situation that resembles the original fall environment with a protective tension response. This response, as described in Chapter One, actually increases fall risk rather than reducing it.

The most effective way to reduce this fear-based tension over time is through graduated re-exposure: returning to the environment where the fall happened, or to environments that resemble it, at a pace and with a support that makes the experience manageable. Each successful navigation of that environment begins to replace the threat memory with a competence memory. The nervous system learns, slowly, that the environment is manageable.

This is not about being brave. It is about understanding what the fear is made of and providing the nervous system with new, more accurate information. The fear says the environment is not safe. The competence memory says the environment is manageable with the right pace and the right skills. The more competence memories accumulate, the quieter the fear becomes.

If you have had a fall recently and are returning to outdoor walking after a period of reduced activity, start in the safest, most familiar environment available to you. A flat, quiet pavement near home during daylight, ideally with a companion on the first few occasions. Do not start by returning to the exact location of the fall. Start where success is most likely and build from there. The program's Week One exercises are the appropriate starting point regardless of how long you have been inactive.

It also helps to be honest with yourself about which environments you have been avoiding since the fall. Not to force yourself back into them immediately, but to have a specific list of what successful re-engagement would look like, so that progress is measurable. When the avoided environment becomes accessible again, you will know. The absence of the hesitation that used to accompany it is the clearest sign that the nervous system has updated its assessment.

SAFETY NOTE:
If you are returning to walking after a fall that resulted in a fracture or hospital admission, please speak with your physiotherapist or doctor before starting this program. Their guidance should take precedence over any general program.

Weather, Lighting, and Outdoor Safety Tips

Cold weather tightens muscles and stiffens joints, both of which reduce the quality of walking mechanics. In cold conditions, always do the warm-up from Chapter Three indoors before going out, not in the open air. Dress in layers that allow free arm movement. Cold, restricted shoulders reduce the arm swing that stabilizes the gait. Gloves that are thin enough to maintain hand sensitivity are better than bulky ones that reduce grip if you need to hold a rail.

Wet and icy conditions are genuinely high-risk for older adults and there is no exercise program that makes them safe to walk on unprepared. In wet conditions, slow down significantly, avoid metal surfaces such as drain covers and manhole lids, and choose the middle of the pavement where puddles and ice are less likely to accumulate than at the edges. In icy conditions, the safest choice is to wait. No errand is worth the risk that ice presents. If you must go out, use the widest possible base of support, keep both hands free, and take very small steps with a deliberate flat-footed contact rather than the usual heel-first.

Lighting matters more than many people realize. Dim or poorly lit environments significantly reduce the visual balance input that helps compensate for reduced proprioception. Carry a small torch in a coat pocket when walking in early morning or evening. Many inexpensive key ring torches are bright enough to illuminate the pavement a few steps ahead without being cumbersome. This single habit prevents a disproportionate number of evening falls.

Walking alone outdoors in Weeks One and Two is fine, but telling someone where you are going and roughly when you plan to return is a sensible precaution that costs nothing. By Weeks Three and Four, most people feel confident enough with the new walking habits that this additional step is less necessary. The decision is yours, and it should be based on honest assessment of how the walking is going rather than on either excessive caution or undue confidence.

Chapter 8

After Day 28 – Keeping the Progress Going

The 28 days are finished. The practice is not. This chapter helps you read the Day 28 results honestly and decide what to do with them.

Reading Your Day 28 Results Honestly

The Day 28 progress check at the end of Chapter Five asked you to compare your walking now to where it was on Day 1. Before you decide anything about what comes next, read those answers back. Not the ones you wanted to give. The ones you actually gave.

Clear improvement across all five check items is the best outcome and it happens for most people who complete the program consistently. The heel lands first more reliably. The balance pause is steadier. The confidence in at least one specific real-world situation has increased. If this is your result, what you have built is real and it is already in the body. The decision that matters now is not what to do next. It is what to protect. The progress will not maintain itself without continued practice.

Partial improvement, clear gains in one or two areas but limited change in others, is also a common outcome and it is not a failure. It tells you exactly where the remaining work is. If the heel landing has improved but the confidence in real-world situations has not yet changed, the physical training has worked and the psychological re-exposure has not yet had enough accumulated evidence to shift the fear response. More repetitions in managed real-world environments will close that gap. If balance improved but the obstacle step-over still feels uncertain, more time specifically on Exercise 10 will address it.

Limited overall improvement after a full 28 days of consistent practice is the least common outcome, and it usually has one of three explanations. The first is incomplete consistency: sessions were missed regularly enough that the neural adaptation could not build. The appropriate response is to run the program again with higher completion. The second is a physical condition that requires medical management alongside the exercise: a vestibular disorder, inner ear problem, or neurological condition that affects balance independently of the training. The appropriate response is medical evaluation. The third is that the baseline assessment was inaccurate, and the improvements exist but are not visible in the comparison. If you feel that your walking has changed but the checklist does not reflect it, trust the feeling and find more specific language for what changed.

Continuing the Program on Your Own Terms

The simplest continuation after Day 28 is to run the program again from Week One. The second run is a qualitatively different experience from the first. The exercises are familiar. The cognitive load of learning new movement patterns is gone. The attention that went into remembering the steps can now go into refining the quality of each one. Most people find the second run produces a deeper, more settled improvement than the first run delivered.

If you do not want to repeat the full 28-day structure, build your own daily practice from the twelve exercises. A ten-minute daily session using any combination of exercises that addresses your current priorities is the maintenance minimum. Use Exercise 12 (Confidence Walk) at the end of every session as a consistent self-check. If the Confidence Walk feels less fluid on a given week than the week before, return to whichever earlier exercises you have been skipping.

The exercises do not have to be done in the order the program uses them. Once you know all twelve, you can sequence them by what you need. On a day when balance has been feeling uncertain, lead with the Step and Pause and the Wide-Base Side Step. On a day when a specific outdoor challenge is coming up, practice the exercises most relevant to it. The program gave you a library. Use it like one.

The one non-negotiable in any continuation is daily practice. The proprioceptive and neural adaptations that this program produces are maintained by continued stimulation. A practice done five days a week produces better maintenance than one done twice a week for a longer duration. Frequency matters more than session length at the maintenance stage. Ten minutes daily keeps the gains. Two forty-minute sessions per week simply does not produce the same result.

Adding More Distance, Speed, or Challenge

More distance, meaning longer outdoor walks beyond the ten to twelve minute sessions, can be added from Week Five onward if the Day 28 results showed clear improvement in all three main areas. Start with an additional five minutes of ordinary walking added to the end of the daily session. Increase by five minutes per week. The standard for adding distance is not how far you feel like going. It is whether the heel-to-toe mechanics remain intact throughout the extended walk. If the mechanics deteriorate after fifteen minutes, the additional distance is currently beyond the capacity you have built.

Speed should increase only when balance at the current pace is fully reliable. This is a later development than most people expect. Many people who complete the program find that their walking speed has already increased slightly as a natural result of the improved mechanics, without any deliberate effort to speed up. If your natural walking pace has returned toward something closer to what it was five or ten years ago, that is the right kind of speed increase. Deliberately walking faster to feel more normal is a different thing and it bypasses the proprioceptive reading that the slower pace provides.

A useful self-test for readiness to add speed or distance: perform Exercise 12 (Confidence Walk) for two full minutes at your current normal pace. If the heel landing is fully automatic and the balance feels solid throughout, your mechanics are ready for more challenge. If either element requires active attention to maintain, continue at the current level for another week before reassessing.

New challenges can be added progressively: more complex outdoor routes, steeper slopes, busier environments, less familiar pavements. The principle for adding challenge is the same as the principle for the program: do not add a challenge that cannot be managed with good mechanics at a deliberate pace. If a new surface or environment requires you to rush or to hold constant tension to manage it, it is too advanced for now. Return to it after more practice time.

Walking for the Long Run

The factor that determines whether this program's gains persist for months and years, or whether they fade within weeks of finishing, is not how hard you worked during the 28 days. It is whether the daily practice continues after them.

Daily habits are maintained by structure, not by motivation. Motivation is variable. It is high when the practice is new, when improvement is rapid, or when a specific goal is clear. It is low when the practice has become familiar, when improvement has plateaued, or when the day is full of other demands. Building the walking practice into a fixed daily structure, a specific time, a specific location, a consistent opening sequence, removes the motivational decision. The practice occurs because the structure calls for it, not because motivation happened to be available.

The morning is the most effective time for this practice, for the same reason that Chapter Three recommends morning sessions: the joints are at their stiffest, the cortisol awakening response is naturally anti-inflammatory, and the session positions the rest of the day's walking mechanics favorably. A morning practice is also more protected from disruption than an afternoon or evening one, which tends to get displaced by the accumulation of daily demands.

The most durable version of this practice is one that requires the fewest decisions to maintain. The shoes by the door. The same ten minutes each morning. The same starting point. The same three closing breaths. The repetition of the context is the repetition of the habit. Each time the structure is followed, the neural pathway that makes following it automatic is strengthened.

There will be disruptions: travel, illness, family demands, bad weather. The response to disruption that protects the habit best is returning to practice on the first available day, starting with Week One exercises regardless of how long the break was, and not treating the disruption as a reset that requires starting over emotionally. The body retains more of the training than you expect after a break. The mechanics come back faster the second time, because the neural pathways that built them are still there, just quieter. The habit, if the structure is maintained, does not require rebuilding from scratch.

The walk that feels safe, confident, and effortless is not a destination. It is the daily product of a practice that is simple enough to maintain, short enough to sustain, and specific enough to keep producing the results that make maintaining it genuinely worthwhile over years. Ten minutes. Every day. That is the whole prescription.

Did You Find This Book Quite Helpful?

If it did, then that's worth something and deserves a place on Amazon.

A short review on Amazon takes two minutes and costs nothing. But for an independent author with no marketing budget, it means everything. It is how the next reader finds this book. It is how a daughter finds the right gift for her aging mother and father. It is how this work continues to reach the people it was made for.

Search ***Tai Chi Walking Exercises for Seniors Over 60 by Liuhe Chen*** on Amazon. One or two honest sentences is all it takes.

Thank you for reading. It was an honor to take this trip with you.

Conclusion

What the 28 Days Actually Built

Preventing falls is not achieved by being more careful. It is achieved by having a body that responds more reliably when something unexpected happens underfoot. The heel-first landing habit, the toe-lift on every step, the deliberate pause in Step and Pause, all of these have been building the specific neural pathways that manage the fraction of a second between a stumble and a fall. Whether those pathways are faster and more reliable than they were on Day 1 is something only you can know, from the evidence of the past 28 sessions. But the training was specific, the repetitions were consistent, and the nervous system responds to that.

Rebuilding balance is a slow process and 28 days is enough time to begin it, not to complete it. What the program built is a foundation: stronger outer hip stabilizers from the side-stepping work, better upper ankle coordination from the heel-to-toe and precision walking, and a proprioceptive system that has been deliberately challenged and exercised rather than left to decline. That foundation will hold and continue to develop as long as the practice continues. The balance you have on Day 28 is better than the balance you had on Day 1, and the balance you will have on Day 56 is available to be better still.

Walking with confidence is the outcome that tends to surprise people most, because it shows up in small and specific ways rather than all at once. The kerb that no longer requires a pause to calculate. The car park that felt manageable last week in a way it would not have before. The staircase descended without the hand gripping the rail as tightly. These small moments are the program's real results. They are the practical, daily expression of everything the exercises were building.

The Walk That Belongs to You

The safest, most independent version of your walking is not a fixed standard to reach. It is a moving target that your practice keeps pace with. The body changes over time. The practice adapts with it. An older adult who has maintained a daily walking practice for five years is not in the same physical condition as someone who completed a 28-day program once. They are in an ongoing relationship with their walking capacity that keeps the gap between current ability and current challenge manageable.

The exercises in this program are not complicated. They are specific. The specificity is what makes them effective. Generic walking does not train the heel-landing habit. Generic exercise does not build the outer hip stabilizers that prevent a sideways fall. Generic activity does not practice the backward step or the obstacle clearance that real-world walking requires. These things are built through specific, deliberate, repeated practice of exactly the right movements. You have been doing that for 28 days. That is the difference.

Liuhe has worked with many older adults over the years who came to a walking practice after a fall, after a scare, or after noticing that their confidence had quietly narrowed without them making a deliberate decision to limit themselves. What they found, without exception, was that the capacity for safer, more confident walking had not gone. It had just not been asked for recently. This program asked for it, consistently, for 28 days. The asking is what produced the answer.

Keep the practice. Keep the shoes by the door. Keep the ten minutes. The walk you want is the one you take every day with a little more attention than the day before. That is all this has ever been.

About the Author

Liuhe Chen has practiced Tai Chi for over twenty years. Most of that time has been spent teaching older adults, many of whom had never tried anything like it before and were not sure their bodies were up to it.

Some came after a fall. Some came on doctor's advice. Some came because a friend dragged them along and they ended up staying. Whatever brought them through the door, most of them had one thing in common: they wanted to feel steadier, stronger, and more confident in their own body. That is what Liuhe has spent two decades helping people achieve.

The teaching has always been simple. No complicated moves. No pressure to keep up. Just gentle, steady practice that meets people where they are, whether that means sitting in a chair, moving slowly through joint pain, or starting from scratch after years of little activity. Liuhe has worked with people in their seventies, eighties, and beyond, and has seen again and again that age is not the obstacle most people assume it is.

This book grew out of all those years of working with real people in real situations. It is written for anyone who wants to move better, feel better, and age on their own terms.

Liuhe practices every morning, rain or shine, and still finds something new in it each time.